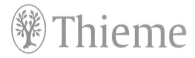

Neurosurgery Primary Examination Review

High Yield Questions, Answers, Diagrams, and Tables

Amgad S. Hanna, MD
Associate Professor
Department of Neurological Surgery
University of Wisconsin School of
   Medicine and Public Health
Madison, Wisconsin

227 illustrations

Thieme
New York • Stuttgart • Delhi • Rio de Janeiro

Executive Editor: Timothy Hiscock
Managing Editor: Apoorva Goel
Director, Editorial Services: Mary Jo Casey
Production Editor: Shivika
International Production Director: Andreas
    Schabert
International Marketing Director: Fiona Henderson
Editorial Director: Sue Hodgson
International Sales Director: Louisa Turrell
Senior Vice President and Chief Operating Officer:
    Sarah Vanderbilt
President: Brian D. Scanlan

Library of Congress Cataloging-in-Publication Data
Names: Hanna, Amgad S., author.
Title: Neurosurgery primary examination review :
high yield questions, answers, diagrams, and tables /
Amgad S. Hanna.
Description: New York : Thieme, [2019] | Includes
bibliographical references and index.
Identifiers: LCCN 2018043035| ISBN
9781626234901 (alk. paper) | ISBN 9781626234963
(eISBN)
Subjects: | MESH: Neurosurgical Procedures—
methods | Examination Questions
Classification: LCC RD593 | NLM WL 18.2 | DDC
617.4/80076—dc23 LC record available at https://
lccn.loc.gov/2018043035

© 2019 Thieme Medical Publishers, Inc.
Thieme Publishers New York
333 Seventh Avenue, New York, NY 10001 USA
+1 800 782 3488, customerservice@thieme.com

Thieme Publishers Stuttgart
Rüdigerstrasse 14, 70469 Stuttgart, Germany
+49 [0]711 8931 421, customerservice@thieme.de

Thieme Publishers Delhi
A-12, Second Floor, Sector-2, Noida-201301
Uttar Pradesh, India
+91 120 45 566 00, customerservice@thieme.in

Thieme Publishers Rio de Janeiro,
Thieme Publicações Ltda.
Edifício Rodolpho de Paoli, 25° andar
Av. Nilo Peçanha, 50 – Sala 2508
Rio de Janeiro 20020-906, Brasil
+55 21 3172 2297

Cover design: Thieme Publishing Group
Typesetting by Thomson Digital, India

Printed in USA by King Printing Company, Inc.
                                    5 4 3 2 1

ISBN 978-1-62623-490-1

Also available as an e-book:
eISBN 978-1-62623-496-3

Important note: Medicine is an ever-changing science undergoing continual development. Research and clinical experience are continually expanding our knowledge, in particular our knowledge of proper treatment and drug therapy. Insofar as this book mentions any dosage or application, readers may rest assured that the authors, editors, and publishers have made every effort to ensure that such references are in accordance with **the state of knowledge at the time of production of the book**.

Nevertheless, this does not involve, imply, or express any guarantee or responsibility on the part of the publishers in respect to any dosage instructions and forms of applications stated in the book. **Every user is requested to examine carefully** the manufacturers' leaflets accompanying each drug and to check, if necessary in consultation with a physician or specialist, whether the dosage schedules mentioned therein or the contraindications stated by the manufacturers differ from the statements made in the present book. Such examination is particularly important with drugs that are either rarely used or have been newly released on the market. Every dosage schedule or every form of application used is entirely at the user's own risk and responsibility. The authors and publishers request every user to report to the publishers any discrepancies or inaccuracies noticed. If errors in this work are found after publication, errata will be posted at www.thieme.com on the product description page.

Some of the product names, patents, and registered designs referred to in this book are in fact registered trademarks or proprietary names even though specific reference to this fact is not always made in the text. Therefore, the appearance of a name without designation as proprietary is not to be construed as a representation by the publisher that it is in the public domain.

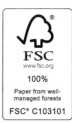

Dear neurosurgery resident,

This book is dedicated to you, current learner and soon-to-be colleague. I don't want you to struggle as much as I once struggled to prepare for the written boards. The books available today are great resources but have a lot of knowledge gaps. This book is not meant to be a full textbook of neurosurgery, but to fill-in some of those knowledge gaps, while presenting the information in a concise and easy-to-remember format. I hope, and am sure, it will make your studying easier, more pleasant, and most importantly more efficient.

Wishing you the best in your endeavors.

Contents

Contents

Foreword

Amgad S. Hanna has provided young neurosurgeons with a review of multiple scientific topics in neurosurgery, organized clearly into the major topics of anatomy, pathology, neurobiology, radiology, critical care, neurology, and neurosurgery. It provides a concise review of these topics for the resident in training or neurosurgery graduate wishing to review these topics. The tables and study sections help organize the material in a thoughtful manner. In addition, the content is presented in the form of questions with answer keys that provide important information regarding the appropriate differentials. I think many will find this book a handy way to organize their thoughts to review the major topics of neurosurgery and a useful study guide in preparation for both exams and academic review.

Robert J. Dempsey, MD
Chairman and Manucher Javid Professor of
Neurological Surgery
Department of Neurological Surgery
University of Wisconsin SMPH
Madison, Wisconsin
Chairman, Foundation for International
Education in Neurological Surgery
Co-Chairman, Coordinating Committee for
International Initiatives for the WFNS

Foreword

It is a special pleasure and rare privilege for me to write the introduction for this book by Dr. Amgad S. Hanna, a peripheral nerve fellow of mine in 2009, to christen it symbolically. As a strong proponent of board review courses, I have long recognized, appreciated, and admired Amgad's unwavering commitment to resident education, training, and development.

This book is clearly a labor of love. In its infancy, some of the materials were used as a hidden secret, a local product available at his home program (University of Wisconsin, Madison). Because of internal success and encouragement, 4 years (and, I suspect, more than 10,000 hours) later, it has morphed into this treasure chest, ripe with countless pearls, and ready for wider use and distribution.

This book differs from other available references for the American Board of Neurological Surgery primary examination. In addition to 20 chapters with 10 tests and 600 questions with self-explanatory answers, it proudly and prominently features two other practical sections with more than 30 diagrams and over 30 tables. This combination of different modalities will help students not only learn but imbibe facts in a practical, efficient, and self-directed fashion.

In my opinion, this review book should be both on the shelves of all neurosurgical residents and also in their pockets, as they prepare for their board examination(s) and for their future career.

Robert J. Spinner, MD
Chairman, Department of Neurologic Surgery
Burton M. Onofrio, MD Professor of Neurosurgery
Professor of Orthopedics and Anatomy
Mayo Clinic
Rochester, Minnesota

Preface

After writing *Anatomy and Exposures of Spinal Nerves and Nerve Cases,* I felt the need to write a book targeting neurosurgery residents studying for their primary (written) board examination. The material is largely from the common review books and textbooks. It also incorporates some of the keywords provided by the American Board of Neurological Surgery. It is in a multiple-choice questions (MCQs format. Each chapter contains 60 questions covering two or three topics, with two chapters dedicated to comprehensive tests. Only one answer is correct. This is a collection of tests that were provided as an in-service to the residents at the University of Wisconsin. Their scores correlated highly with their scores on the actual test. There was also noticeable improvement as they did more practice tests. I recommend that the candidates study the topics first from their preferred sources and then take the test and time themselves. Each test should take less than an hour to answer.

The supplemental material in the last two sections of the book contains high-yield information in the form of concise tables and illustrative diagrams. The diagrams are unique and were all designed by the author. The references are limited to landmark papers and are listed in a nontraditional way under their corresponding answer explanations. For the learner, it is convenient to make the argument for the answer, and I highly recommend downloading the original papers as PDFs and keeping on file for more in-depth study of the topic.

I believe that between the questions, tables, and diagrams, this book will be an essential part of the study armamentarium for written boards. It is not meant to replace other traditional books but to fill in the knowledge gaps and help with self-assessment. The figures and tables are uniquely designed to help present the information in a way that is easy to memorize. I wish you the best in your studies.

Amgad S. Hanna, MD

Acknowledgments

The author would like to thank Dr. Shahriar Salamat for providing some of the histological pictures and their interpretations; Drs. Gregory D. Avey, Beverly L. Aagaard-Kienitz, David B. Niemann, Kimberly Hamilton, and Andrew Scarano for providing some cases; Drs. Ulas Cikla and Omer S. Sahin for helping with the brain sections; and Ms. Barbara Hanna and Mrs. Linda Hanna for editing the book for English language.

Abbreviations

5-HT	serotonin (5-hydroxytryptamine)	ETV	endoscopic third ventriculostomy
a	artery	GCS	Glasgow Coma Score
ABG	arterial blood gas	GFAP	glial fibrillary acid protein
Ach	acetylcholine	GP	globus pallidus
ACOM	anterior communicating artery	Hb	hemoglobin
ACTH	adrenocorticotropic hormone	Hrs	hours
ADC	apparent diffusion coefficient	ICA	internal carotid artery
ADEM	acute disseminated encephalomyelitis	ICP	intracranial pressure
ADH	antidiuretic hormone	ICU	intensive care unit
ADP	adenosine diphosphate	IJV	internal jugular vein
AICA	anterior inferior cerebellar artery	INO	internuclear ophthalmoplegia
AIN	anterior interosseous nerve	IV	intravenous
ASA	acetyl salicylic acid (Aspirin)	LE	lower extremity
ATP	adenosine triphosphate	MAP	mean arterial blood pressure
AVM	arteriovenous malformation	MCA	middle cerebral artery
BBB	blood brain barrier	MEP	motor evoked potentials
BG	basal ganglia	MLF	medial longitudinal fasciculus
B/L	bilateral	Mo	months
CAD	coronary artery disease	MRA	magnetic resonance angiography
CCK	cholecystokinin	MRI	MR imaging
CK	creatine kinase	MSH	melanocyte-stimulating hormone
CNS	central nervous system	MVC	motor vehicle collision
COPD	chronic obstructive pulmonary disease	MVD	microvascular decompression
CSF	cerebrospinal fluid	n	nerve
CT	computerized tomography	NASCET	North American Symptomatic Carotid Endarterectomy Trial
CTA	CT angiography	NE	norepinephrine
DBS	deep brain stimulation	NF1	neurofibromatosis type 1
DNET	dysembryoplastic neuroepithelial tumor	NF2	neurofibromatosis type 2
Ds	days	NMDA	N-methyl-D-aspartate
DSA	digital subtraction angiography	NSAIDs	non-steroidal anti-inflammatory drugs
ECA	external carotid artery	PCA	posterior cerebral artery
EEG	electroencephalogram	PCOM	posterior communicating artery
EMA	epithelial membrane antigen	PICA	posterior inferior cerebellar artery
EMG	electromyography	PIN	posterior interosseous nerve
Enk	enkephalin	PNET	primitive neuroectodermal tumor
ER	emergency room	RBCs	red blood corpuscles
ESR	erythrocyte sedimentation rate	SAH	subarachnoid hemorrhage
ETOH	alcohol		

SC	spinal cord		UE	upper extremity
SEGA	Subependymal giant cell astrocytoma		v	vein
SN	substantia nigra		VGCC	voltage-gated calcium channels
SRS	stereotactic radiosurgery		VMA	vanillylmandelic acid
SSEP	somatosensory evoked potentials		WHO	World Health Organization
STN	subthalamic nucleus		Wks	weeks
tPA	tissue plasminogen activator		Yrs	years

Section I.   Questions and Answers

-

1 Test 1—Anatomy and Neurology

1.
All of the following are characteristics of Wallenberg's syndrome, *except*

A. Ipsilateral Horner's syndrome
B. Vertebral artery occlusion
C. Ipsilateral decreased pain and temperature in the body
D. Ipsilateral ataxia
E. Ipsilateral decreased pain and temperature in the face

2.
Antibodies to presynaptic voltage-gated Ca^{++} channels (VGCC), in patients with oat cell lung carcinoma are associated with

A. Stiff-man syndrome
B. Lambert–Eaton myasthenic syndrome
C. Myasthenia gravis
D. Anti-Hu antibodies
E. Anti-Yo antibodies

3.
Struthers ligament is associated with entrapment of

A. Median n at the elbow
B. Median n at the wrist
C. Ulnar n at the elbow
D. Ulnar n at the wrist
E. Radial n

4.
A 65-year-old male had transient aphasia and was found to have 75% ICA stenosis. The ideal treatment is

A. Observation and treatment of risk factors
B. Daily Aspirin 81 mg
C. Daily Aspirin 325 mg
D. IV heparin followed by oral Coumadin
E. Carotid endarterectomy

5.
The yearly risk of rupture of cerebral AVM is

A. 0–1%
B. 1–2%
C. 2–4%
D. 4–6%
E. 6–8%

6.
All of the following statements are true regarding the cerebellar climbing fibers, *except*

A. They arise in the contralateral inferior olivary nucleus
B. They traverse the inferior cerebellar peduncle
C. They climb to the molecular layer
D. They synapse with the stellate and basket cells
E. They inhibit Purkinje cells

7.
What is the typical location for endoscopic third ventriculostomy (ETV)?

A. Anterior to the optic chiasm
B. Between the chiasm and the pituitary infundibulum
C. Between the median eminence and the mammillary bodies
D. Just posterior to the mammillary bodies
E. None of the above

8.
The most common location for a saccular brain aneurysm is

A. Anterior communicating a (ACOM)
B. Posterior communicating a (PCOM)
C. Middle cerebral a (MCA)
D. Basilar a tip
E. Posterior inferior cerebellar a (PICA)

9.
A 25-year-old male presents with daily unilateral headache associated with rhinorrhea, lacrimation, and conjunctival injection. The most likely diagnosis is

A. Classic migraine
B. Migraine variant
C. Tension headache
D. Cluster headache
E. Pseudotumor cerebri

10.

In the following diagram, the thalamostriate v is labeled

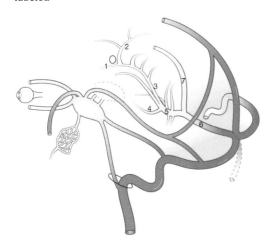

A. 1
B. 2
C. 3
D. 4
E. 5

11.

In the above diagram, the basal v of Rosenthal is labeled

A. 3
B. 4
C. 5
D. 6
E. 7

12.

The yearly risk of rupture of cavernous malformations of the brain is

A. 0.5–1%
B. 1–2%
C. 2–4%
D. 4–6%
E. 6–8%

13.

Venous hypertension (Foix–Alajouanine syndrome) is found in which type(s) of spinal AVMs?

A. Type I
B. Type II
C. Type III
D. Types II and III
E. Types I and IV

14.

Neurofibrillary tangles and neuritic plaques are histologic features of

A. Huntington's chorea
B. Pick's disease
C. Alzheimer's disease
D. Wilson's disease
E. Parkinson's disease

15.

Which cranial nerves are involved in Collet–Sicard syndrome?

A. III and IV
B. V and VI
C. VII and VIII
D. IX, X, XI, and XII
E. None of the above combinations

16.

Parkinson's disease is primarily caused by degeneration of cells in

A. Subthalamic nucleus
B. Substantia nigra
C. Corpus striatum
D. Globus pallidus externus
E. Globus pallidus internus

17.

Meralgia paresthetica causes pain and numbness in the

A. Medial thigh
B. Anterolateral thigh
C. Medial leg
D. Anterolateral leg
E. Sole of foot

18.

Hypsarrhythmia on EEG occurs in which syndrome?

A. Lennox–Gastaut syndrome
B. Absence seizures
C. Grand mal epilepsy
D. Night terrors
E. West syndrome

19.

The main neurotransmitter of the climbing fibers is

A. Glutamate
B. GABA
C. Acetylcholine
D. 5-HT
E. Substance P

20.

The proatlantal a

A.   Is located between the occiput and C1
B.   Is located between C1 and C2
C.   Passes through the hypoglossal canal
D.   Is found in the internal auditory canal
E.   Connects ICA to ECA

21.

Based on the ISUIA (International Study of Unruptured Intracranial Aneurysms), asymptomatic anterior circulation aneurysms should be treated if equal to or greater than

A.   2 mm
B.   3 mm
C.   5 mm
D.   7 mm
E.   10 mm

22.

The risk of stroke after a TIA over 2 years, in patients with >70% carotid artery stenosis, is

A.   6%
B.   11%
C.   26%
D.   50%
E.   60%

23.

All of the following vessels contribute to the blood supply of the internal capsule, *except*

A.   Anterior choroidal a
B.   PCA
C.   PCOM
D.   Recurrent a of Heubner
E.   Lateral lenticulostriate aa

24.

Normal cerebral blood flow is

A.   <8 mL/100 g/min
B.   8–23 mL/100 g/min
C.   24–49 mL/100 g/min
D.   50 mL/100 g/min
E.   51–100 mL/100 g/min

25.

Internuclear ophthalmoplegia (INO) is associated with all of the following, *except*

A.   Can be caused by multiple sclerosis (MS)
B.   Is caused by lesion of the ipsilateral medial longitudinal fasciculus (MLF)
C.   Causes failure of adduction of the ipsilateral eye
D.   Causes failure of abduction of the contralateral eye
E.   Can be bilateral

26.

Incremental response of compound muscle action potential (CMAP) is observed in

A.   Myasthenia gravis
B.   Lambert–Eaton myasthenic syndrome (LEMS)
C.   Amyotrophic lateral sclerosis (ALS)
D.   Myotonia congenita
E.   Anti-Hu antibodies

27.

The daily production of cerebrospinal fluid (CSF) is about

A.   75 mL
B.   150 mL
C.   300 mL
D.   450 mL
E.   600 mL

28.

At the ischemic penumbra, the cerebral blood flow is

A.   <8 mL/100 g/min
B.   8–23 mL/100 g/min
C.   24–49 mL/100 g/min
D.   50 mL/100 g/min
E.   51–100 mL/100 g/min

29.

The blood–brain barrier (BBB) is intact within which structure?

A.   Neurohypophysis
B.   Pineal gland
C.   Area postrema
D.   Subfornical organ
E.   Subcommissural organ

30.

The tentorial a is a branch of which segment of the ICA?

A. Cervical
B. Petrous
C. Lacerum
D. Intracavernous
E. Supraclinoid

31.

An autosomal recessive disorder characterized by accumulation of phytanic acid is

A. Refsum's disease
B. Niemann–Pick's disease
C. Hurler's disease
D. Morquio's syndrome
E. Krabbe's disease

32.

Early subacute blood appears hyperintense on T1- and hypointense on T2-weighted MRI due to

A. Oxyhemoglobin
B. Deoxyhemoglobin
C. Intracellular methemoglobin
D. Extracellular methemoglobin
E. Hemosiderin

33.

Wave V of the brainstem auditory evoked responses (BAERs) represents activation of

A. Cochlear nuclei
B. Superior olivary nucleus
C. Lateral lemniscus
D. Inferior colliculus
E. Auditory radiation

34.

After a subarachnoid hemorrhage, when a patient is lethargic and confused with no focal deficits, the Hunt and Hess grade is

A. I
B. II
C. III
D. IV
E. V

35.

A cerebral AVM of 3.5 cm in diameter, in the dominant temporal lobe, and with deep venous drainage, corresponds to which Spetzler–Martin grade?

A. I
B. II
C. III
D. IV
E. V

36.

The lesion marked by the *arrows* in the following MRI will most likely cause

A. Subarachnoid hemorrhage
B. Gelastic seizures
C. Absence seizures
D. Panhypopituitarism
E. Metastasis

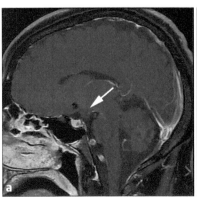 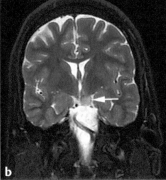 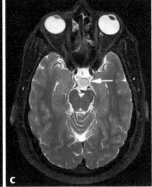

37.

Which of the following is true about the anatomy of the spinal cord?

A. In the topographic representation of the posterior columns, the legs are medial.
B. In the lateral corticospinal tract, the legs are medial.
C. In the lateral spinothalamic tract, the legs are medial.
D. Fine touch and proprioception travel in the lateral funiculus.
E. In the anterior horn, the appendicular muscles are medial.

38.

The main neurotransmitter in the substantia gelatinosa of Rolando is

A. Glutamate
B. GABA
C. Acetylcholine
D. Dopamine
E. Substance P

39.

The pterion is located at the junction of all of the following bones, *except*

A. Frontal
B. Zygoma
C. Greater wing of sphenoid
D. Squamous temporal
E. Parietal

40.

Bill's bar separates

A. Facial n from superior vestibular n
B. Facial n from cochlear n
C. Superior from inferior vestibular nerves
D. Cochlear n from inferior vestibular n
E. Facial n from inferior vestibular n

41.

Somnambulism occurs in which stage of sleep?

A. REM (rapid alternating eye movements)
B. 1
C. 2
D. 4

42.

Nightmares occur in which stage of sleep?

A. 1
B. 2
C. 3
D. 4
E. REM (rapid alternating eye movements)

43.

A 41-year-old female was involved in a motor vehicle accident. She was positive for alcohol, amphetamines, and tricyclic antidepressants. Her injuries included closed head injury (CT head below, see **a**), minor rib fractures, and liver laceration. Initial examination revealed that she was neurologically intact. Five days later, she developed confusion and right hemiparesis. Angiogram is shown below. The most likely cause of her symptoms is

A. Blossomed contusion
B. Fat embolism
C. Cardio-embolic
D. Carotid dissection
E. Carotid atherosclerosis

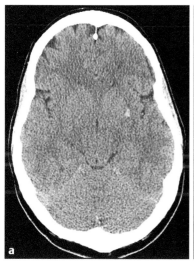
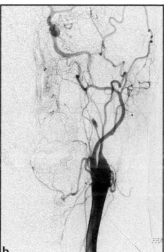
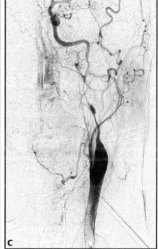

44.

Thoracic disc herniation patients are *least* likely to improve after which surgical approach?

A.   Endoscopic transthoracic
B.   Open transthoracic
C.   Laminectomy
D.   Transpedicular
E.   Costotransversectomy

45.

A trauma that leads to Chance fracture, usually involves

A.   Flexion only
B.   Flexion and distraction
C.   Extension and distraction
D.   Axial load
E.   Axial rotation

46.

Froment's test is used to depict

A.   Median neuropathy
B.   Ulnar neuropathy
C.   Radial neuropathy
D.   Tenosynovitis
E.   Rheumatoid arthritis

47.

All of the following structures enter the orbit through the annulus of Zinn, *except*

A.   Oculomotor n, superior division
B.   Oculomotor n, inferior division
C.   Trochlear n
D.   Nasociliary n
E.   Abducens n

48.

Nervi erigentes provides

A.   Somatic supply to the genitals
B.   Sympathetic supply to the genitals
C.   Parasympathetic supply to the genitals
D.   Somatic supply to the inner thigh
E.   None of the above

49.

The parasympathetic component of the third cranial nerve arises from

A.   Edinger–Westphal nucleus
B.   Central nucleus
C.   Medial nucleus
D.   Lateral nucleus
E.   Superior salivary nucleus

50.

Taste sensation of the anterior 2/3 of tongue is carried by

A.   Trigeminal n
B.   Chorda tympani n
C.   Glossopharyngeal n
D.   Vagus n
E.   None of the above

51.

The thalamic nucleus that receives input from the globus pallidus and projects to the premotor and supplementary motor cortices is

A.   Medial dorsal (MD)
B.   Lateral dorsal (LD)
C.   Ventral Anterior (VA)
D.   Ventrolateral pars caudalis (VLc)
E.   Ventrolateral pars oralis (VLo)

52.

The cortical area that connects mostly with the lateral posterior (LP) nucleus of thalamus is

A.   Frontal lobe
B.   Parietal lobe
C.   Occipital lobe
D.   Temporal lobe
E.   Cingulate gyrus

53.

The large pyramidal cells occupy which layer of the cerebral cortex?

A.   I
B.   II
C.   III
D.   IV
E.   V

54.

The uncinate fasciculus connects

A.   Orbito-frontal gyri to anterior temporal lobe
B.   Anterior temporal lobe to occipital lobe
C.   Orbito-frontal gyri to parietal lobe
D.   Parietal to occipital lobe
E.   Frontal, parietal, parahippocampal, and temporal

55.
The corticobulbar fibers occupy which part of the internal capsule?

A. Anterior limb
B. Genu
C. Posterior limb
D. Retrolenticular
E. Sublenticular

56.
In the following figure, the subiculum is represented by number

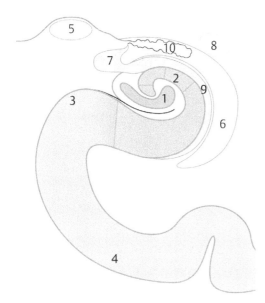

A. 1
B. 2
C. 3
D. 4
E. 5

57.
In the above figure, the fimbria is represented by number

A. 1
B. 2
C. 3
D. 5
E. 7

58.
What is a contraindication to an anterior odontoid screw?

A. Age > 50
B. Fracture line horizontal
C. Fracture line oblique downward and posteriorly
D. Very large barrel chest
E. Inability to open the mouth > 2 cm

59.
The superior salivary nucleus provides parasympathetic supply that travels through the

A. Facial n
B. Glossopharyngeal n
C. Vagus n
D. All of the above
E. None of the above

60.
The stria terminalis connects

A. The substantia nigra to the caudate nucleus
B. The amygdala to the hypothalamus
C. The hypothalamus to the salivary nuclei
D. The amygdala to the nucleus accumbens septi
E. The lateral hypothalamus to the hippocampus

2 Answer Key 1

1.

C Ipsilateral decreased pain and temperature in the body

Wallenberg's (lateral medullary) syndrome is caused by vertebral a or PICA (posterior inferior cerebellar artery) occlusion. The clinical picture is ipsilateral except for pain and temperature in the body, which is contralateral (ventral and lateral spinothalamic tracts) (**Fig. 13E**).

2.

B Lambert–Eaton myasthenic syndrome

Lambert–Eaton myasthenic syndrome is characterized by antibodies to presynaptic voltage-gated Ca⁺⁺ channels (VGCC). Myasthenia gravis is caused by antibodies to nicotinic AChR (acetylcholine receptors) or MuSK (muscle-specific kinase). Anti-Hu is associated with lung cancer (oat cell carcinoma) and lymphoma. Anti-Yo is associated with ovarian and breast cancer. Stiff-man (Moersch–Woltman) (Stiff-person) syndrome is related to anti-GAD (glutamic acid decarboxylase) is non-paraneoplastic, or anti-amphiphysin or anti-gephyrin which are paraneoplastic (**Table 16**).

3.

A Median n at the elbow

The liga*m*ent of Struthers can attach to a *m*edial supracondylar process of the hu*m*erus and cause entrapment of the *m*edian n proximal to the elbow joint. The arcade of Struthers (controversial) can be associated with ulnar n entrapment at the elbow and may cause recurrence after decompression. The posterior interosseous n (PIN), a branch of the radial nerve can be entrapped under the arcade of Fröhse.

4.

E Carotid endarterectomy

According to NASCET (North American Carotid Endarterectomy Trial), carotid endarterectomy reduces the risk of stroke for symptomatic carotid artery stenosis of ≥70%, from 26% to 9% at 2 years.

Further Reading: North American Symptomatic Carotid Endarterectomy Trial Collaborators. Beneficial effect of carotid endarterectomy in symptomatic patients with high-grade carotid stenosis. *N Engl J Med.* 1991;325:445–453

5.

C 2–4%

The annual risk of rupture of cavernomas is 0.5–1%, aneurysms 1–2%, and AVMs 2–4%.

6.

E They inhibit Purkinje cells

The climbing (olivocerebellar) fibers are excitatory secreting glutamate. Also, mossy fibers and granule cells are excitatory. Purkinje cells are inhibitory.

7.

C Between the median eminence and the mammillary bodies

Endoscopic third ventriculostomy is performed in the floor of the third ventricle between the *M*ammillary bodies and the *M*edian eminence (**Fig. 23**).

8.

A Anterior communicating a (ACOM)

Incidence of saccular aneurysms of the brain:

ACOM: 40%

PCOM: 30%

MCA: 20%

Basilar: 8%

PICA: 2%

9.

D Cluster headache

Typical description of cluster headache: young adult male, unilateral headache, parasympathetic discharge causing lacrimation, rhinorrhea, and conjunctival injection. It occurs every day for weeks to months.

10.

B. 2

1. Septal v, 2. thalamostriate v, 3. internal cerebral v, 4. basal v of Rosenthal, 5. v of Galen, 6. straight sinus, 7. inferior sagittal sinus (**Fig. 5**).

11.

B 4

12.

A 0.5–1%

The annual risk of rupture of cavernous malformations is 0.5–1%, aneurysms 1–2%, and AVMs 2–4%.

13.

E Types I and IV

Spinal AVMs types I and IV are high flow, low pressure, they present with venous hypertension; while types II and III are high flow, high pressure, they present with hemorrhage (**Table 17**).

14.

C Alzheimer's disease

Histologic characteristics of neurodegenerative diseases. Alzheimer's: neurofibrillary tangles and neuritic plaques; Huntington's: caudate atrophy; Pick's: Pick bodies; Wilson's: Opalski cells; and Parkinson's: Lewy bodies (**Table 14**).

15.

D IX, X, XI, and XII

Collet–Sicard syndrome is a unilateral lower cranial nerves palsy (IX, X, XI, and XII) usually caused by trauma or tumors (**Table 15**).

16.

B Substantia nigra

Parkinson's disease is caused by failure of dopaminergic output from the substantia nigra pars compacta to the corpus striatum. Hemiballismus is caused by lesions of the subthalamic nucleus. Huntington's chorea, manganese, and methanol toxicity affect the striatum. Athetosis has involvement of the globus pallidus externus, while carbon monoxide and manganese affect the globus pallidus internus (**Fig. 7**).

17.

B Anterolateral thigh

Meralgia paresthetica is caused by entrapment or injury of the lateral femoral cutaneous n; it causes pain and numbness in the anterolateral thigh. The medial thigh is supplied by the ilioinguinal n, femoral n, and obturator n, medial leg by the saphenous n (a branch of the femoral n), anterolateral leg by the peroneal n, and the sole of the foot by the medial and lateral plantar nn (branches of the tibial).

18.

E West syndrome

West syndrome is characterized by hypsarrhythmia on EEG: large bilateral slow waves with multifocal spikes; Lennox–Gastaut: spike-dome 1–2 Hz; absence: spike-dome 3 Hz; juvenile myoclonic epilepsy: spike-dome 4–6 Hz; grand mal: repetitive spikes up to 100 **μ**V. Night terrors occur in stages 3 and 4 of non-REM sleep (**Fig. 31**).

19.

A Glutamate

Climbing fibers consist of the olivocerebellar tract, which travels within the inferior cerebellar peduncle. Together with the granule cells, they synapse with Purkinje cell dendrites in the molecular cell layer, are excitatory, and secrete glutamate. Mossy fibers are also excitatory but end in the granular layer (**Fig. 11**).

20.

A Is located between the occiput and C1

The proatlantal a is an anastomosis between the vertebral a and either the internal or external carotid a (ICA or ECA); it travels between the occiput and C1. The hypoglossal a connects the ICA to the basilar a and travels through the hypoglossal canal. The acoustic (otic) a connects the ICA to the basilar a through the internal auditory canal.

21.

D 7 mm

Based on the ISUIA study, the risk of rupture of asymptomatic anterior circulation aneurysms, excluding PCOM, <7 mm is very low.

Further Reading: Wiebers DO, Whisnant JP, Huston J 3rd, et al.; International Study of Unruptured Intracranial Aneurysms Investigators. Unruptured intracranial aneurysms: natural history, clinical outcome, and risks of surgical and endovascular treatment. *Lancet* 2003 Jul 12;362(9378):103–110

22.

C 26%

Based on NASCET (North American Symptomatic Carotid Endarterectomy Trial), carotid endarterectomy reduces the risk of stroke from 26% to 9% over 2 years in symptomatic patients with 70–99% stenosis, or 50–69% in high risk patients.

Further Reading: North American Symptomatic Carotid Endarterectomy Trial Collaborators. Beneficial effect of carotid endarterectomy in symptomatic patients with high-grade carotid stenosis. *N Engl J Med.* 1991;325:445–453

23.

B PCA

The internal capsule is supplied by the anterior choroidal, PCOM, Heubner, and lateral lenticulostriate aa (**Fig. 6**). The PCA does not contribute to the blood supply of the internal capsule.

24.

D 50 mL/100 g/min

The normal cerebral blood flow is 50 mL/100 g/min, with higher flow in the gray matter than the white matter. In the ischemic penumbra, it is 8–23 mL/100 g/min. The normal Oxygen consumption is 3.5 mL/100 g/min.

25.

D Causes failure of abduction of the contralateral eye

INO causes failure of the ipsilateral eye to adduct due to a lesion of the MLF (medial longitudinal fasciculus). Failure to abduct is caused by VI n palsy and not INO.

26.

B Lambert–Eaton myasthenic syndrome (LEMS)

LEMS is caused by antibodies against presynaptic VGCC. It is associated with oat cell pulmonary carcinoma and is characterized by incremental response of CMAP.

27.

D 450 mL

The normal adult CSF volume is 150 mL, of which 30 mL is intraventricular, 40 mL spinal subarachnoid space, and 80 mL cranial subarachnoid space. The body produces 3 times the CSF volume per day (450 mL).

28.

B 8–23 mL/100 g/min

The ischemic penumbra is at 8–23 mL/100 g/min of cerebral blood flow. EEG is isoelectric <18 mL/100 g/min. At 12 mL/100 g/min, there is failure of Na^+/K^+ ATPase. Irreversible damage occurs <8 mL/100 g/min.

29.

E Subcommissural organ

The subcommissural organ is the only circumventricular organ with intact BBB (**Fig. 24B**).

30.

D Intracavernous

The tentorial artery of Bernasconi and Cassinari is a branch of the meningohypophyseal trunk of the intracavernous carotid a. The meningohypophyseal trunk also gives the dorsal meningeal and inferior hypophyseal. The intracavernous carotid a also gives the McConnell's capsular a and the inferior cavernous a.

31

A Refsum's disease

Refsum's disease is autosomal recessive, caused by phytanic acid oxidase deficiency, characterized by retinitis pigmentosum, deafness, cardiomyopathy, and peripheral neuropathy (sensory-motor, symmetric, predominantly in the lower extremities) (**Table 13**).

32.

C Intracellular methemoglobin

In the early subacute stage (3–14 ds), intracellular metHb appears bright (hyperintense) on T1- and dark (hypointense) on T2-weighted MRI (**Table 5**).

33.

D Inferior colliculus

BAERs waves: I: cochlear n; II: cochlear nuclei; III: superior olivary nucleus; IV: lateral lemniscus; V: inferior colliculus; VI: medial geniculate body; VII: auditory radiation (**Fig. 31**).

34.

C III

Based on the main features of the Hunt and Hess grading system for subarachnoid hemorrhage: grade I: mild headache, II: severe headache or cranial nerve deficits, III: lethargy, IV: hemiparesis, V: extensor posturing (**Table 22**).

35.

D 4

Based on the Spetzler-Martin grading system, the presented AVM is 3-6 cm (2), in an eloquent cortex (1), and with deep venous drainage (1). Therefore, this patient's AVM is grade IV (**Table 20**). The higher the grade, the higher the surgical morbidity.

36.

B Gelastic seizures

Hypothalamic hamartomas (*arrows*) cause gelastic seizures.

37.

A In the topographic representation of the posterior columns, the legs are medial.

In the spinal cord, the arms are lateral in the posterior columns (cuneate tract); these transmit fine touch and proprioception. The arms are medial in the spinothalamic and lateral corticospinal tracts. In the anterior horn, the axial muscles are medial while the appendicular muscles are lateral and the extensor muscles are ventral while the flexor muscles are dorsal (**Fig. 15**).

38.

E Substance P

The substantia gelatinosa of Rolando is represented by layer II of the Rexed laminae in the posterior horn of the spinal cord. It transmits pain and utilizes substance P as its neurotransmitter (**Fig. 15**).

39.

B Zygoma

The pterion is H-shaped and is made of: frontal, parietal, squamous part of temporal bone, and the greater wing of the sphenoid bone.

40.

A Facial n from superior vestibular n

In the internal acoustic meatus, the facial n is above the cochlear n (7-up, coke down), the superior vestibular n is above the inferior vestibular n, and the facial n is medial to the superior vestibular n and separated from it by the Bill's bar (**Fig. 14**).

41.

D 4

Somnambulism, night terrors, and enuresis are associated with stages 3 and 4 of sleep (**Fig. 31**).

42.

E REM (rapid alternating eye movements)

Nightmares and sleep apnea occur during REM sleep. Nocturnal epilepsy occurs during stage 4 or REM sleep (**Fig. 31**).

43.

D Carotid dissection

The patient suffered a left carotid dissection as evidenced by the smooth tapering of the left ICA (*arrow*) and the pseudoaneurysm (*arrowhead*). She did not respond to therapeutic anticoagulation. She then underwent successful stenting under barbiturate burst suppression.

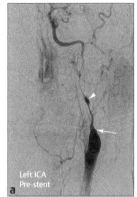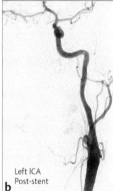

Left ICA Pre-stent

a

Left ICA Post-stent

b

44.

C Laminectomy

Thoracic disc herniation can be successfully treated by a transpedicular, transfacet, costotransversectomy, lateral extracavitary, or transthoracic approaches. Laminectomy has a high risk of worsening.

45.

B Flexion and distraction

Chance fracture is usually caused by a flexion and distraction (seat-belt) injury.

46.

B Ulnar neuropathy

Froment's test is performed by asking the patient to hold on to a piece of paper between the thumb and index fingers using adductor pollicis which is supplied by the ulnar n. In case of ulnar n palsy, as the examiner tries to pull on the paper, the patient flexes the distal phalanx of the thumb using flexor pollicis longus supplied by the AIN (median n).

47.

C Trochlear n

Structures entering the orbit outside the annulus of Zinn are: LFT: Lacrimal n (from V_1), Frontal n (from V_1), Trochlear n (IV), in addition to the superior ophthalmic vein.

48.

C Parasympathetic supply to the genitals

Nervi erigentes (pelvic splanchnic nn; S2,3,4) provide parasympathetic supply to the pelvis and perineum.

49.

A Edinger -Westphal nucleus

Edinger–Westphal nucleus provides parasympathetic component of the oculomotor n (III) (general visceral efferent). The general somatic efferents arise from the central nucleus supplying levator palpebrae superioris bilaterally, medial nucleus supplying contralateral superior rectus, and lateral nucleus supplying ipsilateral inferior rectus, inferior oblique, and medial rectus. The superior division supplies levator palpebrae superioris and superior rectus. The parasympathetic fibers occupy the outside of III and are more vulnerable to compressive lesions, like PCOM aneurysms (**Fig. 14**).

50.

B Chorda tympani n

While somatic sensation of the anterior 2/3 of the tongue (general somatic afferents) is supplied by V, taste sensation (special visceral afferents) is provided by the chorda tympani branch of VII. The posterior 1/3 of the tongue is supplied by IX for both somatic and taste sensations (**Fig. 14**).

51.

E Ventrolateral pars oralis (VLo)

VLo (Voa) receives afferents from GP and projects to premotor cortex. VLc and VPLo receive afferents from the dentate nucleus and projects to motor area 4. VA receives input from SN, areas 6 and 8 and projects to premotor cortex. MD receives input from prefrontal cortex, temporal cortex, amygdala, SN, and GP and projects to prefrontal cortex. LD sends projections to the cingulate gyrus (**Fig. 8**).

52.

B Parietal lobe

LP nucleus of thalamus has sensory projections to the parietal lobe, areas 5 and 7 (**Fig. 8**).

53.

E V

In a 6-layer cortex model, the main output from the internal pyramidal layer (V) is to the brain stem and spinal cord, and from the multiform layer (VI) to the thalamus. The main afferents connect to the internal granular layer (IV). The molecular (I), external granular (II), and external pyramidal (III) layers connect to other cortical areas, while III connects the 2 hemispheres (**Fig. 3**).

54.

A Orbito-frontal gyri to anterior temporal lobe

The uncinate fasciculus connects orbito-frontal gyri to anterior temporal lobe. The arcuate fasciculus connects the superior and middle frontal gyri to the temporal lobe. The superior longitudinal fasciculus: frontal to parietal and occipital. The inferior longitudinal fasciculus: temporal to occipital.

55.

B Genu

The corticobulbar fibers occupy the genu of the internal capsule, corticospinal the posterior half of the posterior limb with the legs represented posteriorly, auditory projections in sublenticular, visual in retrolenticular. The anterior limb contains the anterior thalamic peduncle (**Fig. 6**).

56.

C 3

1, Dentate gyrus; 2, Cornu Ammonis (hippocampus); 3, subiculum; 4, entorhinal cortex; 5, optic tract; 6, temporal horn of lateral ventricle; 7, fimbria of fornix; 8, tail of caudate nucleus; 9, alveus; 10, choroid plexus (see also **Fig. 4**).

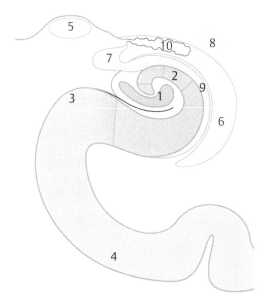

57.

E 7

58.

D Very large barrel chest

Barrel chest will preclude the ability to get the appropriate trajectory for an odontoid screw. A fracture line oblique downward and anteriorly will not allow purchase in the broken fragment. Inability to open the mouth is a contraindication for a transoral approach for odontoidectomy.

59.

A Facial n

The superior salivary nucleus provides parasympathetic efferents (general visceral efferents) through the chorda tympani branch of the facial n to the submandibular and sublingual salivary glands, through the greater superficial petrosal n to the lacrimal gland. The inferior salivary nucleus provides parasympathetic efferents to the glossopharyngeal n (parotid gland) and the dorsal vagal nucleus to the vagus n (**Fig. 14**).

60.

B The amygdala to the hypothalamus

The stria terminalis connects the hypothalamus and septal nuclei to the amygdala. The stria medullaris provides efferents from the septal nuclei to the habenular nuclei (**Figs. 9 and 10**).

3 Test 2—Pathology, Radiology, and Critical Care

1.

The following section is characteristic of which brain tumor?

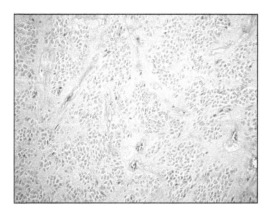

A. Medulloblastoma
B. Ependymoma
C. Pineoblastoma
D. Retinoblastoma
E. Hemangiopericytoma

2.

Which of the following is *not* a feature of Duchenne's muscular dystrophy?

A. Autosomal recessive inheritance
B. Increased serum creatine kinase
C. Positive Gower's test
D. Muscle fiber necrosis and regeneration
E. Congestive heart failure

3.

Ryanodine receptor mutation occurs in

A. Mitochondrial myopathies
B. Kearns–Sayre syndrome
C. Familial periodic paralysis
D. Malignant hyperthermia
E. Acute intermittent porphyria

4.

Phytanic acid oxidase deficiency causes

A. Phenylketonuria
B. Sandhoff's disease
C. Refsum's disease
D. Fabry's disease
E. Hurler's disease

5.

A 64-year-old female presents with paraparesis, decreased sensation in the lower extremities, and no pain, the most likely diagnosis is:

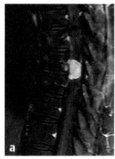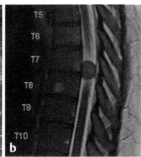

A. Nerve sheath tumor
B. Drop metastasis
C. Hemangiopericytoma
D. Myxopapillary ependymoma
E. Meningioma

6.

The optic n fibers have their cell of origin from

A. The ganglion cells
B. Amacrine cells
C. Bipolar cells
D. Horizontal cells
E. Photoreceptor cells (rods and cones)

7.

The best treatment for torsade de pointes is

A. 3% saline infusion
B. 1.8% saline infusion
C. Normal saline
D. Magnesium sulfate infusion
E. Potassium chloride infusion

8.

All of the following are characteristics of tuberous sclerosis, *except*

A. Autosomal dominant inheritance on chromosome 17
B. Subependymal giant cell astrocytoma (SEGA)
C. Cardiac rhabdomyoma
D. Renal angiolipoma
E. Liver cysts

9.

The following lesion was removed from the temporal lobe of a 10-year-old boy with seizures. What is the diagnosis?

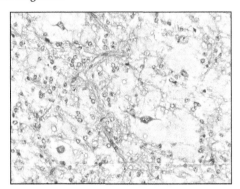

A. Ganglioglioma
B. Dysembryoplastic neuroepithelial tumor (DNET)
C. Oligodendroglioma
D. Central neurocytoma
E. Glioblastoma multiforme

10.

A 64-year-old man undergoes an angiogram for embolization of a posterior fossa mass prior to surgical resection. What anatomical variation (*arrow*) is observed in the following ECA angiogram?

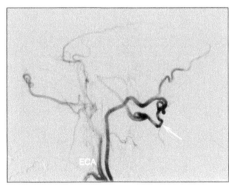

A. Fetal PCOM a
B. Persistent primitive trigeminal a
C. Persistent primitive otic a
D. Persistent primitive hypoglossal a
E. Persistent primitive proatlantal a

11.

Based on the previous angiogram, which vascular structure is identified by the *arrow*?

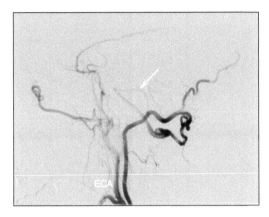

A. PICA
B. AICA
C. PCA
D. Superior cerebellar a
E. Vertebral a

12.

The metabolic disorder inherited as autosomal recessive, characterized by α L-iduronidase deficiency, mental retardation, gargoyle face, thick meninges, spinal cord compression, and zebra bodies is called

A. Hurler's disease
B. Hunter's syndrome
C. Gaucher's disease
D. Tay–Sachs disease
E. Morquio's syndrome

13.

Which of the following is *not* an inclusion criterion for neurofibromatosis type 2 (NF2)?

A. Bilateral vestibular schwannomas
B. Positive family history
C. Sphenoid dysplasia
D. Postcapsular cataract
E. Meningioma

14.

Gum hyperplasia, hirsutism, ataxia, thrombocytopenia, and Stevens–Johnson syndrome can all occur with which anti-epileptic drug?

A. Ethosuximide
B. Valproic acid
C. Carbamazepine
D. Phenytoin
E. Phenobarbital

15.

The lesion at T9-T10 depicted in the following figure could be safely removed through all of the following approaches, *except*

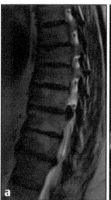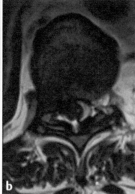

A.   Thoracotomy
B.   Thoracoscopy
C.   Costotransversectomy
D.   Transpedicular
E.   Laminectomy

16.

The nuclear bag intrafusal fibers have which of the following feature

A.   Eccentric in position
B.   Flower-spray endings
C.   Type Ia fibers conducting at 70–120 m/s
D.   Are smaller than the nuclear chain fibers
E.   Have a static response

17.

Which drug could be complicated by cyanide toxicity?

A.   Nitroglycerin
B.   Sodium nitroprusside
C.   Norepinephrine
D.   Dopamine
E.   Dobutamine

18.

At what gestational date does the posterior neuropore close?

A.   16 days
B.   18 days
C.   22 days
D.   24 days
E.   28 days

19.

Which receptor transmits vibration sensation?

A.   Pacinian corpuscle
B.   Hair end organ
C.   Ruffini end organ
D.   Merkel's disc
E.   Free nerve endings

20.

The abnormality depicted in this MRI occurs at which gestational age?

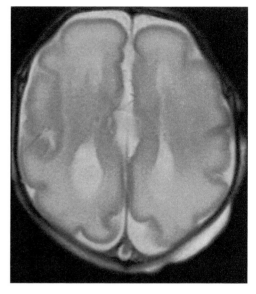

A.   3–4 weeks
B.   4–5 weeks
C.   5–10 weeks
D.   2–5 months
E.   5–9 months

21.

Warfarin (Coumadin) level is increased by all of the following drugs, *except*

A.   Phenobarbital
B.   Salicylates
C.   Bactrim
D.   Cimetidine
E.   Benzodiazepines

22.

Orogenital ulcers, uveitis, ulcerative colitis, erythema nodosum, polyarthritis, and confusion could all occur in

A.   Takayasu's arteritis
B.   Wegener's granulomatosis
C.   Buerger's disease
D.   Behçet's disease
E.   Cogan's syndrome

23.

Superoxide dismutase mutation causes

A. McArdle's disease
B. Amyotrophic lateral sclerosis (ALS)
C. Duchenne's muscular dystrophy
D. Werdnig–Hoffmann disease
E. Charcot–Marie–Tooth disease

24.

The lesion depicted in the following figure is from an AIDS patient. It was biopsied and the histology is shown. The most likely diagnosis is

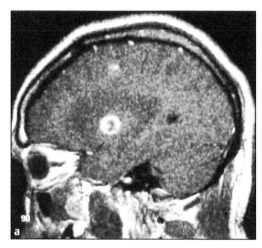

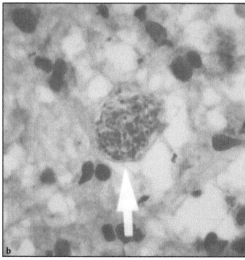

A. Bacterial brain abscess
B. Fungal brain abscess
C. Toxoplasmosis
D. Glioblastoma
E. Multiple sclerosis (MS)

25.

Fibers in the corpus callosum originate in which layer of the cerebral cortex?

A. I
B. II
C. III
D. V
E. VI

26.

The Golgi tendon organ sends signals through which of these fibers?

A. Ia
B. Ib
C. II
D. III
E. IV

27.

Which of the following drugs is a specific α1 receptor blocker?

A. Prazosin
B. Clonidine
C. Guanethidine
D. Reserpine
E. Labetalol

28.

Basophilic stippling of red blood corpuscles is caused by which toxicity?

A. Methotrexate
B. Cisplatin
C. Arsenic
D. Mercury
E. Lead

29.

Which autosomal recessive disease is caused by N-acetyl-aspartoacylase deficiency and causes mental retardation, macrocephaly, and blindness?

A. Krabbe's disease
B. Adrenoleukodystrophy
C. Pelizaeus–Merzbacher disease
D. Canavan's disease
E. Cockayne's syndrome

30.

The following sections are from a temporal lobe lesion in a patient with seizures, what is the diagnosis?

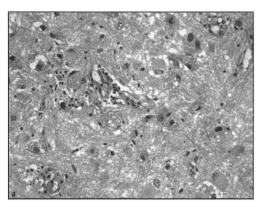

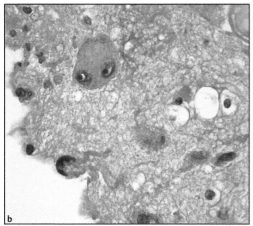

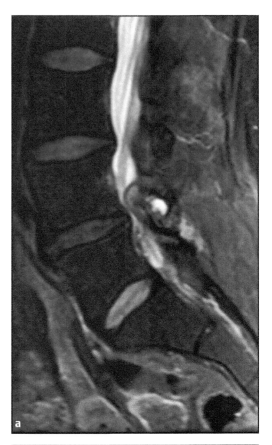

A. Lymphoma
B. Oligodendroglioma
C. Ganglioglioma
D. Dysembryoplastic neuroepithelial tumor (DNET)
E. Giant cell astrocytoma

31.

A 63 year old female with left L5 radiculopathy, has the following MRI, the most likely diagnosis is:

A. Extruded left L4-L5 disc fragment
B. Synovial cyst
C. Cystic schwannoma
D. Arachnoid cyst
E. Osteoid osteoma

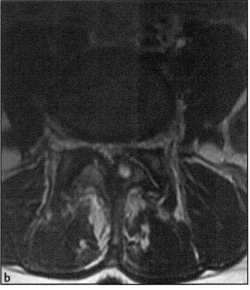

32.

Muscarinic acetylcholine receptors are found at the

A. Neuromuscular junction
B. Preganglionic endings of sympathetic fibers
C. Postganglionic endings of most sympathetic fibers
D. Preganglionic endings of parasympathetic fibers
E. Postganglionic endings of parasympathetic fibers

33.

Which drug has no β2 agonist effect?

A. Phenylephrine (Neosynephrine)
B. Epinephrine
C. Isoproterenol
D. Dobutamine
E. Dopamine

34.

Which disease causes cherry-red spot in the macula, hepatosplenomegaly, and mental retardation and is caused by sphingomyelinase deficiency?

A. Gaucher's disease
B. Fabry's disease
C. Niemann–Pick's disease
D. Maple syrup urine disease
E. Hunter's disease

35.

For a 58-year-old male with bilateral lower extremity pain has the following MRI. What is the most likely diagnosis?

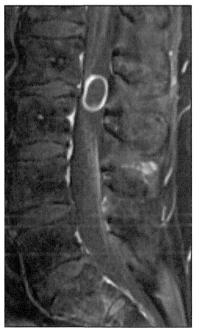

A. Hemangioblastoma
B. Drop metastasis
C. Meningioma
D. Schwannoma
E. Neurofibroma

36.

The following tumor was removed from the cerebellopontine angle of a patient. What is the diagnosis?

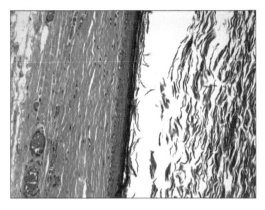

A. Meningioma
B. Vestibular schwannoma
C. Dermoid cyst
D. Epidermoid cyst
E. Metastasis

37.

High anion gap acidosis can be caused by all of the following, *except*

A. Renal tubular acidosis
B. Diabetic ketoacidosis
C. Lactic acidosis
D. Methanol
E. Salicylate toxicity

38.

Spike-dome waves at 3 Hz on an EEG are characteristic of

A. Stage 3 of sleep
B. Absence seizures
C. Generalized seizures
D. West syndrome
E. REM sleep

39.

What is a DNA repair disorder characterized by CNS and peripheral nerve demyelination, cataract, and dwarfism?

A. Maroteaux–Lamy syndrome
B. Sandhoff's disease
C. Alexander's disease
D. Lowe's syndrome
E. Cockayne's syndrome

40.

Increased urine δ-aminolevulinic acid (δ-ALA) occurs in

A. Kearns–Sayre syndrome
B. Familial periodic paralysis
C. Acute intermittent porphyria
D. Malignant hyperthermia
E. Central core disease

41.

What type of tumor is depicted below?

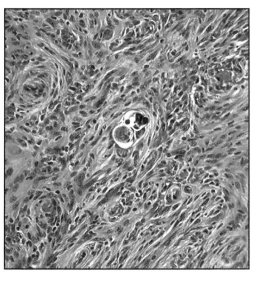

A. Schwannoma
B. Glioblastoma
C. Meningioma
D. Metastasis
E. Chordoma

42.

The following is a picture of a newborn. This disorder is caused by failure of

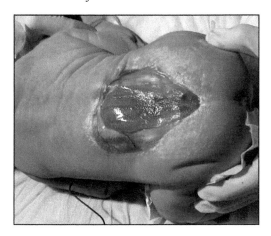

A. Primary neurulation
B. Secondary neurulation
C. Disjunction
D. Ventral induction
E. Migration

43.

Which disease is autosomal recessive, caused by decreased liver peroxisomes, with long-chain fatty acid accumulation, and a cerebro-hepato-renal syndrome?

A. Lowe's syndrome
B. Zellweger's syndrome
C. Leigh's disease
D. Lesch–Nyhan disease
E. Alexander's disease

44.

The following extra-axial tumor was very hemorrhagic during resection. What is the most likely diagnosis?

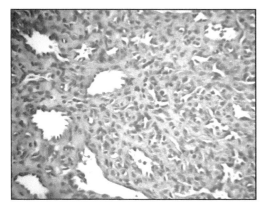

A. Chordoma
B. Meningioma
C. Hemangioblastoma
D. Hemangiopericytoma
E. Chondrosarcoma

45.

The following tumor is observed in which syndrome?

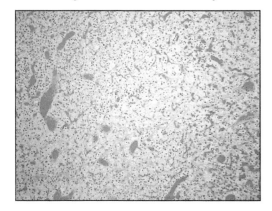

A. Von Hippel–Lindau syndrome
B. Tuberous sclerosis
C. Neurofibromatosis type 1
D. Neurofibromatosis type 2
E. Gorlin's syndrome

46.

Which of the following is an autosomal dominant disorder caused by a genetic defect in coding for calcium in muscle fiber membranes and results in paralysis when exposed to cold weather or exercise?

A. Mitochondrial myopathy
B. Kearns–Sayre syndrome
C. Familial periodic paralysis
D. Malignant hyperthermia
E. Central core disease

47.

A 38-year-old female presented with headache and vertigo and was found to have the following abnormality on head CTA. What is the *arrow* pointing at?

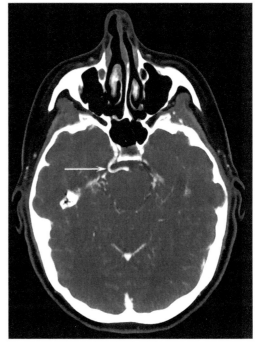

A. Trigeminal schwannoma
B. PCOM
C. Anterior choroidal a
D. Tentorial a of Bernasconi and Cassinari
E. Persistent trigeminal a

48.

The medial forebrain bundle connects

A. Septal nuclei to hippocampus
B. Subiculum to mammillary nuclei
C. Mammillary nuclei to midbrain
D. Lateral hypothalamic nuclei to amygdala
E. Lateral hypothalamic nuclei to septal nuclei

49.

The following histology is seen in which intracranial tumor?

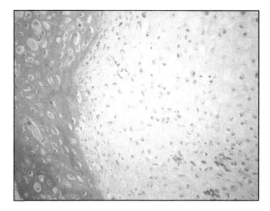

A. Oligodendroglioma
B. Chordoma
C. Meningioma
D. Hemangiopericytoma
E. Hemangioblastoma

50.

Which artery is causing the blush in the following angiogram?

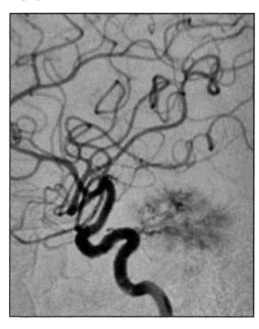

A. Artery of Bernasconi and Cassinari
B. Persistent trigeminal a
C. Vidian a
D. Inferior hypophyseal a
E. McConnell's capsular a

51

Which of the listed eye signs correspond to the NF2 disease?

A. Kayser-Fleischer ring in the cornea
B. Glaucoma
C. Lisch nodules in the iris
D. Postcapsular cataract
E. AVM of the retina and optic nerve

52

Which of the listed eye signs correspond to Wilson's disease?

A. Kayser-Fleischer ring in the cornea
B. Glaucoma
C. Lisch nodules in the iris
D. Postcapsular cataract
E. AVM of the retina and optic nerve

53

Which of the listed eye signs correspond to Wyburn-Mason disease?

A. Kayser-Fleischer ring in the cornea
B. Glaucoma
C. Lisch nodules in the iris
D. Postcapsular cataract
E. AVM of the retina and optic nerve

54

Which of the listed eye signs correspond to the NF1 disease?

A. Kayser-Fleischer ring in the cornea
B. Glaucoma
C. Lisch nodules in the iris
D. Postcapsular cataract
E. AVM of the retina and optic nerve

55

Which of the listed eye signs correspond to the Sturge-Weber syndrome?

A. Kayser-Fleischer ring in the cornea
B. Glaucoma
C. Lisch nodules in the iris
D. Postcapsular cataract
E. AVM of the retina and optic nerve

56.

Which of the following syndromes correspond to Polyostotic fibrous dysplasia?

A. Fahr's disease
B. McCune -Albright syndrome
C. Hallervorden -Spatz disease
D. Von Hippel -Lindau disease
E. Sturge -Weber syndrome

57.

Which of the following syndromes correspond to Bilateral basal ganglia hypodensities?

A. Fahr's disease
B. McCune -Albright syndrome
C. Hallervorden -Spatz disease
D. Von Hippel -Lindau disease
E. Sturge -Weber syndrome

58.

Which of the following syndromes correspond to Tram track appearance on CT?

A. Fahr's disease
B. McCune -Albright syndrome
C. Hallervorden -Spatz disease
D. Von Hippel -Lindau disease
E. Sturge -Weber syndrome

59.

Which of the following syndromes correspond to Bilateral basal ganglia calcifications?

A. Fahr's disease
B. McCune -Albright syndrome
C. Hallervorden -Spatz disease
D. Von Hippel -Lindau disease
E. Sturge -Weber syndrome

60.

Which of the following syndromes correspond to Cystic lesion with a mural enhancing nodule?

A. Fahr's disease
B. McCune -Albright syndrome
C. Hallervorden -Spatz disease
D. Von Hippel -Lindau disease
E. Sturge -Weber syndrome

4 Answer Key 2

1.

B Ependymoma

Ependymomas are characterized by **p**seudorosettes (built around **b**lood vessels). Flexner–Wintersteiner rosettes have a central canal and may occur in ependymoma, retinoblastoma, or pineoblastoma. Homer–Wright rosettes have neither blood vessels nor central canal in the center and are seen in medulloblastoma or PNET. Pineocytomas have very large rosettes (**Table 7**).

2.

A Autosomal recessive inheritance

Duchenne's muscular dystrophy is X-linked recessive, with decreased dystrophin, atrophy shoulder and pelvic girdles, calf pseudohypertrophy, increased CK, and a positive Gower's test. Treatment: prednisone (**Table 13**).

Further Reading: Deconinck N, Dan B. Pathophysiology of Duchenne muscular dystrophy: current hypotheses. *Pediatr Neurol.* 2007 Jan;36(1):1–7

3.

D Malignant hyperthermia

Ryanodine receptor mutation occurs in malignant hyperthermia. Acute intermittent **porph**yria is caused by defective **porph**obilinogen deaminase, familial periodic paralysis by a genetic defect coding for Ca in muscle fiber membranes, Kearns–Sayre syndrome by mitochondrial DNA, non-maternally inherited, and mitochondrial myopathies by maternal mitochondria defect (**Table 13**).

4.

C Refsum's disease

Refsum's disease is caused by phytanic acid oxidase deficiency. It is inherited as autosomal recessive and causes peripheral neuropathy, retinitis pigmentosum, deafness, and cardiomyopathy (**Table 13**).

5.

E. Meningioma

Intradural extramedullary enhancing lesions in postmenopausal females are most likely meningiomas, especially in the thoracic region. Schwannomas are more common in the lumbar spine and cause radicular pain.

6.

A The ganglion cells

The rods and cones transmit the visual signal to the bipolar cells, the latter relay to the ganglion cells, which are the cells of origin of the optic n fibers. Excitation of the photoreceptors results in activation of protein G, 5'GMP, Na^+ channel closure, hyperpolarization, and an electric graded conduction (**Fig. 30**).

7.

D Magnesium sulfate infusion

Torsade de pointes is a serious cardiac dysrhythmia that can be complicated by ventricular fibrillation. It should be promptly treated. Mg is the treatment of choice. An infusion at 3–10 mg/min can be given even if the serum Mg level is normal. Mg decreases Ca influx and suppresses early afterdepolarizations. Other treatments include mexiletine, temporary transvenous ventricular pacing, stopping any offending agents, and correcting electrolyte imbalance. K can be helpful but Mg remains of choice.

8.

A Autosomal dominant inheritance on chromosome 17

Tuberous sclerosis is inherited as autosomal dominant on chromosome 9 (hamartin) or 16 (tuberin). Features include SEGA, facial angiofibroma (adenoma sebaceum), subungual fibroma (Koenen tumor), ash leaf spots, cardiac rhabdomyoma, renal angiolipoma, and liver cysts (**Table 11**).

9.

B Dysembryoplastic neuroepithelial tumor (DNET)

Large neurons floating in mucin, a chicken-wire vascular pattern, small oligodendrocyte-like cells are seen in DNET. Both DNET and ganglioglioma occur in the temporal lobe in children and cause seizures.

10.

E Persistent primitive proatlantal a

Persistent primitive proatlantal a type 2 (*arrow*), corresponds to a segmental artery that connects the external carotid artery to the vertebral a.

11.

A PICA

The vertebral a ends in PICA (*arrow*).

12.

A Hurler's disease

Hurler's disease (MPS IH) features increased urinary dermatan sulfate, zebra bodies, gargoyle face, hepatosplenomegaly, corneal opacities, deafness, mental retardation, and spinal cord compression (**Table 12**).

13.

C Sphenoid dysplasia

Sphenoid dysplasia is a feature of NF1 (**Table 11**).

14.

D Phenytoin

Phenytoin (Dilantin) is a Na channel blocker. It is used for generalized tonic–clonic seizures and status epilepticus. Side effects include rash, Stevens–Johnson syndrome, cerebellar degeneration, diplopia, stupor, peripheral neuropathy, thrombocytopenia, megaloblastic anemia, lymphadenopathy, gum hyperplasia, hirsutism, hepatitis, gastrointestinal irritation, osteopenia, teratogenicity (congenital fetal hydantoin syndrome) (**Table 34**).

15.

E Laminectomy

Laminectomy for thoracic disc herniation carries a high risk of paraplegia.

16.

C Type Ia fibers conducting at 70–120 m/s

Nuclear bag fibers transmit signals through type Ia fibers, while nuclear chain transmit through type II (**Table 3**). A, B, D, and E are also features of nuclear chain.

17.

B Sodium nitroprusside

Sodium nitroprusside can be used in hypertensive emergencies. It may cause cyanide toxicity. Treatment: O_2, nitrites, and thiosulfate (Cyanide Antidote Kit).

18.

E 28 days

During primary neurulation, the neural tube closure starts in the middle at 22 days, then the anterior neuropore at 24 days (lamina terminalis), and then the posterior neuropore at 28 days.

19.

A Pacinian corpuscle

Pacinian and Meissner's corpuscles transmit vibration sense. Touch and pressure are sensed by Ruffini end organs and Merkel's discs. Touch is also sensed by hair end organs and Meissner's corpuscles. Pain is transmitted by free nerve endings (**Table 2**).

20.

D 2–5 months

Agenesis of the corpus callosum and colpocephaly are caused by a defective migration and occur between 2 and 5 months (**Table 9**).

21.

A Phenobarbital

Phenobarbital stimulates hepatic microsomal enzymes and increases degradation of Coumadin. Bactrim, cimetidine, and benzodiazepines inhibit liver enzymes and promote bleeding on Coumadin. Salicylates increase Coumadin level by displacing it from plasma proteins (**Fig. 32**).

22.

D Behçet's disease

Behçet's disease affects small vessels and causes meningo-encephalitis, brain stem edema, confusion, oro-genital ulcers, uveitis, ulcerative colitis, erythema nodosum, polyarthritis. Treatment: corticosteroids (**Table 29**).

23.

B Amyotrophic lateral sclerosis (ALS)

Cu/Zn superoxide dismutase mutation is seen in ALS, myophosphorylase deficiency in McArdle's disease, and decreased dystrophin in Duchenne's muscular dystrophy (**Table 13**).

24.

C Toxoplasmosis

Sagittal MRI with contrast shows the target sign. Histology reveals **b**radyzoites (**b**ound in a **b**ag). These are typical for toxoplasmosis, an opportunistic infection in AIDS patients. Treatment: pyrimethamine + sulfadiazine + leucovorin. Treatment can be started empirically based on clinical suspicion and no biopsy.

25.

C III

Commissural fibers originate in layer III of the cerebral cortex (external pyramidal layer). Ipsilateral cortical connections arise in layers I–III. Layer IV is the main afferent; layer V (internal pyramidal layer) is the main efferent and contains the large pyramidal (Betz) cells. Layer VI sends efferents to the thalamus (**Fig. 3**).

26.

B Ib

Golgi tendon organ sends impulses through Ib (A α) fibers at 120 m/s. It stimulates Renshaw cells to inhibit α motor neurons (**Table 1, Fig. 28**). Renshaw cells utilize the inhibitory neurotransmitter glycine that causes Cl⁻ influx into the neurons. Renshaw cells are inhibited by tetanus and strychnine, causing tetanic contractions (**Figs. 26** and **27**).

27.

A Prazosin

Prazosin, phentolamine, and phenoxybenzamine are α1 receptor blockers; clonidine α2 receptor stimulant, thus decreasing NE release; labetalol α and β blocker. *Reserpine* inhibits *synthesis* and *storage* of NE, while guanethidine inhibits NE release (**Fig. 25**).

28.

E Lead

Basophilic stippling of RBCs occurs in Pb poisoning, cerebellar dysfunction and renal tubular necrosis with Hg, Mees' lines in As, peripheral neuropathy and deafness with cisplatin, and subacute necrotizing leukoencephalitis (SNLE) with methotrexate (**Table 29**).

29.

D Canavan's disease

Metabolic disorders causing macrocephaly include Alexander's, Canavan's, and Tay–Sachs diseases (**Table 12**).

30.

C Ganglioglioma

Perivascular lymphocytes (center in **a**) and large multinucleated ganglion cells (**b**) characterize ganglioglioma. Due to the mixed nature, they are positive for both GFAP and neurofilament.

Calcifications may be observed. They are frequently cystic. They commonly occur in the temporal lobe of children and cause seizures.

31.

B Synovial cyst

Synovial cysts are usually hyperintense on T2 MRI and are associated with the facet joints. When symptomatic, they need to be resected with or without fusion depending on associated instability.

32.

E Postganglionic endings of parasympathetic fibers

Muscarinic acetylcholine receptors are found at the postganglionic endings of parasympathetic fibers as well as postganglionic sympathetic to sweat glands. Nicotinic receptors are in the sympathetic and parasympathetic ganglia, adrenal gland, and the neuromuscular junction (**Figs. 25** and **26**).

33.

A Phenylephrine (Neosynephrine)

Phenylephrine is a vasopressor (α1 stimulation) with no β agonist effects; is a good choice in shock with tachycardia or myocardial infarction. On the other hand, isoproterenol is mainly a β agonist, and epinephrine stimulates both α and β receptors. Dobutamine has very strong β1 inotropic effect and can be used in acute heart failure. Dopamine is also good in cardiogenic shock; it is a positive inotrope (β1), but may cause tachycardia; at low doses, dopamine is vasodilator (β2 and dopaminergic receptors); at high doses vasoconstrictor (α1). Amrinone is a direct inotrope through cAMP (**Table 33, Fig. 25**).

34.

C Niemann-Pick's disease

Lysosomal storage diseases causing a cherry-red spot in the macula are GM1, Sandhoff's, Tay–Sachs (also causes macrocephaly), and Niemann–Pick diseases (**Table 12**).

35.

D Schwannoma

Cystic tumors with enhancing wall in the lumbar spine in males with radicular pain are likely to be cystic schwannomas. The other diagnoses are possible but less common. Meningiomas are more common in the thoracic region in postmenopausal females.

36.

D Epidermoid cyst

Diffuse keratin is typical for epidermoid and dermoid cysts. The absence of hair follicles goes against dermoid. Epidermoids are common in the cerebellopontine angle and show restricted diffusion on MRI.

37.

A Renal tubular acidosis

A metabolic acidosis with high anion gap (AG) is usually caused by organic acid accumulation (unmeasured anions). Normal AG is 12 mEq/L (more recently 3-10 mEq/L). Low AG can be observed in hypoproteinemia. High AG is seen in: **MUD PILES**: methanol, uremia, diabetic ketoacidosis, paracetamol, isoniazid, lactic acidosis (including starvation), ethylene glycol, and salicylates. Renal tubular acidosis is caused by a defect in distal tubule H^+ secretion and/or proximal tubule HCO_3^- absorption causing normal AG metabolic acidosis.

38.

B Absence seizures

Spike-dome waves at 1–2 Hz are seen in Lennox–Gastaut syndrome, 3 Hz in absence seizures, and 4–6 Hz in juvenile myoclonic epilepsy. West syndrome (infantile spasms) is characterized by hypsarrhythmias (**Fig. 31**).

39.

E Cockayne's syndrome

Cockayne's syndrome is a leukodystrophy caused by defective DNA repair (**Table 12**).

40.

C Acute intermittent porphyria

Acute intermittent porphyria is autosomal dominant caused by a defect in porphobilinogen deaminase. The urine has increased delta-ALA and porphobilinogen. It turns dark as it oxidizes. Patients have severe peripheral neuropathy, seizures, psychiatric problems, and abdominal pain. Treatment: hematin (**Table 13**).

41.

C Meningioma

Calcified psammoma body (center) and whorls are characteristics of meningiomas. **Men**ingiomas are positive for **EMA** and vi**men**tin. They can occur with NF2 (chromosome 22).

42.

A Primary neurulation

Myelomeningocele is caused by failure of closure of the neural tube (caudal end normally closes at 28 days). It is a disorder of primary neurulation (**Table 9**).

43.

B Zellweger's syndrome

Zellweger's syndrome is an autosomal recessive disorder, caused by decreased liver peroxisomes, with long-chain fatty acid accumulation, and manifests as a cerebro-hepato-renal syndrome (**Table 12**).

44.

D Hemangiopericytoma

The large staghorn blood vessels are seen in hemangiopericytoma. The tumor is positive for reticulin and vimentin but unlike meningiomas negative for EMA. These tumors tend to be very hemorrhagic and have a high recurrence rate.

45.

A Von Hippel–Lindau syndrome

Hemangioblastomas are rich in blood vessels and clear cells (lipid content). They are positive for vimentin. Unlike renal cell carcinoma, they are negative for EMA and cytokeratin. They are common in the posterior fossa and spinal cord. They can secrete erythropoietin and cause polycythemia. They can be sporadic or part of von Hippel–Lindau syndrome (chromosome 3) (**Table 11**).

46.

C Familial periodic paralysis

Familial periodic paralysis is autosomal dominant disorder caused by genetic defect in coding for calcium in muscle fiber membranes; there is decreased level of serum K. Treatment: KCl, carbonic anhydrase inhibitors (dichlorphenamide), low NaCl, and avoid carbohydrates (**Table 13**).

47.

E Persistent trigeminal a

Persistent trigeminal a connects the ICA (precavernous or proximal cavernous) to the basilar a. It occurs in 0.2% (0.1–0.5%) of angiograms and courses along the Meckel's cave.

48.

E   Lateral hypothalamic nuclei to septal nuclei

The medial forebrain bundle connects the septal nuclei to the lateral hypothalamic nuclei and the latter to the midbrain (ventral tegmental area). The fornix connects the hippocampus to the septal nuclei, mammillary nuclei, and medial hypothalamus. The stria terminalis connects the amygdala to the septal nuclei and lateral hypothalamus. The ventral amygdalofugal fibers also connect the amygdala to the hypothalamus and septal nuclei. The mammillary nuclei connect to the midbrain through the mammillotegmental tract. The stria medullaris connects the septal nuclei to the habenula (**Figs. 9** and **10**).

49.

B   Chordoma

Chrodomas are characterized by physaliphorous cells and a mucinous background. Normal bone is observed on the left. They are common in the sacrum and clivus. The goal of surgery is en bloc resection. Proton beam therapy can be helpful.

50.

A   Artery of Bernasconi and Cassinari

The tentorial a of Bernasconi and Cassinari causes blush in cases of tentorial meningiomas. It is a branch of the meningohypophyseal trunk (from the cavernous ICA), which also gives the dorsal meningeal and inferior hypophyseal aa. The cavernous ICA also gives rise to the McConnell's capsular a and the inferolateral trunk. The vidian and caroticotympanic aa are branches of the petrous ICA. Persistent trigeminal a is very rare and connects ICA to basilar a.

51.

D   Postcapsular cataract

Postcapsular cataract is a feature of NF2 (**Table 11**).

52.

A   Kayser–Fleischer ring in the cornea

Kayser–Fleischer ring occurs in Wilson's disease (**Table 14**).

53.

E   AVM of the retina and optic nerve

Wyburn–Mason disease is characterized by AVM of the retina and optic nerve.

54.

C   Lisch nodules in the iris

Lisch nodules occur in NF1 (**Table 11**).

55.

B   Glaucoma

Glaucoma is a feature of Sturge–Weber syndrome.

56.

B   McCune–Albright syndrome

Polyostotic fibrous dysplasia occurs in McCune–Albright syndrome.

57.

C   Hallervorden–Spatz disease

Hallervorden–Spatz disease features bilateral basal ganglia hypodensities (**Table 14**).

58.

E   Sturge–Weber syndrome

Tram track appearance on CT is seen in Sturge–Weber syndrome due to vascular calcifications.

59.

A   Fahr's disease

Fahr's disease is characterized by bilateral basal ganglia calcifications.

60.

D   Von Hippel–Lindau disease

Cystic lesion with a mural enhancing nodule describes either hemangioblastoma or pilocytic astrocytoma. Neither of these are choices, but the former can occur with von Hippel–Lindau disease (**Table 11**).

5 Test 3—Anatomy and Neurosurgery

1.

Enkephalins are the main neurotransmitters from

A. Cerebral cortex to caudate
B. Subthalamic nucleus to caudate
C. Caudate to putamen
D. Putamen to globus pallidus externus
E. Thalamus to cerebral cortex

2.

Which thalamic nucleus receives mostly input from the cerebellum and has output to the motor cortex?

A. VA (ventral anterior)
B. VLo (ventral lateral, pars oralis) [Voa: ventralis oralis anterior]
C. VLc (ventral lateral, pars caudalis) [Vop: ventralis oralis posterior and Vim: ventralis intermediate nucleus]
D. MD (medial dorsal)
E. LP (lateral posterior)

3.

With basilar tip aneurysm surgery, the highest risk of perforating vessel injury occurs when the aneurysm is directed

A. Anteriorly
B. Posteriorly
C. Cranially
D. To the right
E. To the left

4.

Wartenberg's sign is associated with which nerve injury?

A. Ulnar n
B. Median n
C. Radial n
D. Common peroneal n
E. Tibial n

5.

In the following diagram, the vein of Galen is labeled

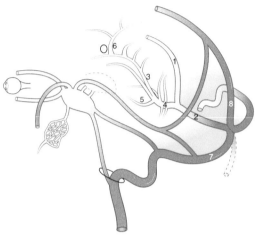

A. 1
B. 2
C. 4
D. 5
E. 7

6.

In the same diagram, the internal cerebral v is labeled

A. 1
B. 3
C. 4
D. 5
E. 6

7.

In the following figure, Ammon's horn is number

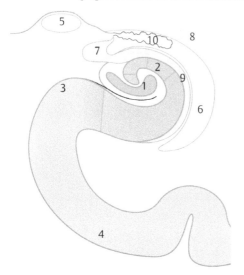

A.   1
B.   2
C.   3
D.   4
E.   7

8.

In the same diagram, the dentate gyrus is number

A.   1
B.   2
C.   3
D.   4
E.   5

9.

During an endoscopic third ventriculostomy, the opening in the floor of the third ventricle should be made

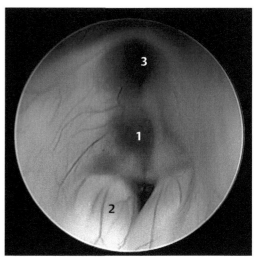

A.   Anterior to 3
B.   Through 3
C.   Through 1
D.   Through 2
E.   Posterior to 2

10.

In the figure above, the infundibular recess is

A.   Anterior to 3
B.   3
C.   1
D.   2
E.   Posterior to 2

11.

The main neurotransmitter from the subthalamic nucleus to the globus pallidus is

A.   Glutamate
B.   Acetylcholine
C.   Dopamine
D.   Serotonin
E.   GABA (Gamma Amino Butyric Acid)

12.
The medial dorsal nucleus of thalamus (MD) projects to the

A.   Prefrontal cortex
B.   Area 4
C.   Areas 3, 1, and 2
D.   Parietal association area
E.   Banks of the calcarine sulcus

13.
In the following view of the foramen of Monro, the fornix is located at

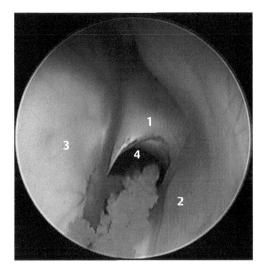

A.   1
B.   2
C.   3
D.   4
E.   None of the above

14.
The corticospinal tract occupies which part of the internal capsule?

A.   Anterior limb
B.   Genu
C.   Anterior part of the posterior limb
D.   Posterior part of the posterior limb
E.   Sublenticular part

15.
In the cerebellar architecture, all of the following structures are inhibitory, *except*

A.   Basket cells
B.   Outer stellate cells
C.   Purkinje cells
D.   Pyramidal cells
E.   Granule cells

16.
The risk of stroke from >70% symptomatic carotid a stenosis at 2 years is

A.   5%
B.   9%
C.   11%
D.   26%
E.   70%

17.
The annual rate of rupture of intracranial aneurysms is

A.   0.5
B.   1–2%
C.   2–4%
D.   6%
E.   20%

18.
The meningohypophyseal trunk is a branch of which segment of the ICA?

A.   Petrous
B.   Cavernous
C.   Clinoidal
D.   Ophthalmic
E.   Communicating

19.
The normal cerebral blood flow is

A.   <8 mL/100 g/min
B.   8–23 mL/100 g/ min
C.   50 mL/100 g/min
D.   75 mL/100 g/min
E.   >75 mL/100 g/min

20.
Which circumventricular organ is paired and enduces emesis?

A.   Subforniceal organ
B.   Subcommissural organ
C.   Organum vasculosum
D.   Area postrema

21.
The cerebrospinal fluid (CSF) is normally produced at a rate of

A.   150 mL/d
B.   300 mL/d
C.   450 mL/d
D.   600 mL/d
E.   750 mL/d

22.

The superior hypophyseal a is a branch of which segment of the ICA?

A.   Petrous
B.   Cavernous
C.   Clinoidal
D.   Ophthalmic
E.   Communicating

23.

The anterior choroidal a supplies all of the following, *except*

A.   Optic tract
B.   Internal capsule
C.   Thalamus
D.   Red nucleus
E.   None of the above

24.

Which artery, when present, is a branch of the P1 segment of the PCA and supplies the thalamus and midbrain bilaterally?

A.   Percheron
B.   Benasconi and Cassinari
C.   Adamkiewicz
D.   Calcarine
E.   Medial posterior choroidal

25.

The proatlantal a connects

A.   The ICA to the ECA
B.   The ICA to the PCA
C.   The petrous carotid a to the basilar a
D.   The cervical carotid a to the basilar a
E.   The cervical carotid a to the vertebral a

26.

According to Lorente de No, the corticospinal tract starts in which layer of the cerebral cortex?

A.   Layer I
B.   Layer II
C.   Layer III
D.   Layer IV
E.   Layer V

27.

The uncinate fasciculus connects

A.   Orbital frontal gyri to anterior temporal lobe
B.   Superior and middle frontal gyri to temporal lobe
C.   Occipital to temporal lobes
D.   Frontal to parieto-occipital lobes
E.   Frontal and parietal to parahippocampal and temporal lobes

28.

The corticospinal tract has 40% of its fibers from

A.   Pyramidal cells of Betz
B.   Area 4
C.   Area 6
D.   Parietal cortex

29.

The thalamic nucleus targeted for DBS to treat tremors is

A.   VA (ventral anterior)
B.   Vim (ventralis intermediate)
C.   Voa (ventralis oralis anterior)
D.   Vop (ventralis oralis posterior)
E.   MD (medial dorsal)

30.

The main neurotransmitter from the substantia nigra to basal ganglia is

A.   Dopamine
B.   GABA: gamma aminobutyric acid
C.   Serotonin
D.   Enkephalins
E.   Glutamate

31.

The rehemorrhage rate after an untreated ruptured cerebral aneurysm in the first 6 months is

A.   5%
B.   10%
C.   20%
D.   50%
E.   80%

32.

If a patient is lethargic and confused after sub-arachnoid hemorrhage, he is Hunt and Hess grade

A. 1
B. 2
C. 3
D. 4
E. 5

33.

A cerebral AVM of 5 cm in diameter, involving the visual cortex, with deep venous drainage, has a surgical risk of major deficit of

A. 4%
B. 7%
C. 12%
D. 19%
E. 69%

34.

The most effective treatment of cranial subdural empyema is

A. Observation
B. Multiple lumbar punctures
C. Antibiotics alone
D. Treat the primary source
E. Surgical evacuation

35.

The pterion is formed by all of the following bones, *except*

A. Frontal
B. Parietal
C. Squamous temporal
D. Greater wing of sphenoid
E. Zygoma

36.

Which of the following is *not* true about the special visceral afferent fibers of the facial n?

A. They transmit taste sensation from the anterior 2/3 of the tongue.
B. They travel through the chorda tympani n.
C. They reach the tongue through the lingual branch of the mandibular division of the trigeminal n.
D. They synapse in the caudal part of the nucleus of tractus solitarius.

37.

All of the following muscles are typically supplied by the median n in the hand, *except*

A. Adductor pollicis
B. Abductor pollicis brevis
C. Flexor pollicis brevis
D. Opponens pollicis
E. The lateral 2 lumbrical muscles

38.

The oculomotor n supplies all of the following muscles, *except*

A. Superior rectus
B. Superior oblique
C. Inferior rectus
D. Inferior oblique
E. Medial rectus

39.

Which of the following nerves enters the orbit outside the annulus of Zinn?

A. Abducens n
B. Nasociliary branch of the ophthalmic division of the trigeminal n
C. Trochlear n
D. Superior division of oculomotor n
E. Inferior division of oculomotor n

40.

Bill's bar separates which 2 nerves?

A. Cochlear and inferior vestibular
B. Cochlear and facial
C. Facial and superior vestibular
D. Facial and inferior vestibular
E. Cochlear and superior vestibular

41.

Which ligament is the cranial extension of the posterior longitudinal ligament (PLL)?

A. Apical ligament
B. Alar ligament
C. Transverse atlantal ligament
D. Membrana tectoria
E. Anterior atlanto-occipital membrane

42.

Which tract of the spinal cord conveys contralateral pain and temperature sensation?

A. Ventral spinothalamic
B. Lateral spinothalamic
C. Ventral spinocerebellar
D. Dorsal spinocerebellar
E. Fasciculus gracilis

43.

When considering the Rexed laminae of the gray matter of the spinal cord, substance P is the main neurotransmitter in layer

A. II
B. IV
C. VI
D. VII
E. IX

44.

The arcade of Struthers can be associated with entrapment of the

A. Musculocutaneous n
B. Median n
C. Ulnar n
D. Radial n
E. Peroneal n at the fibular neck

45.

Froment's sign is positive with paralysis of the

A. Interossei
B. Flexor pollicis longus
C. Flexor pollicis brevis
D. Abductor pollicis brevis
E. Adductor pollicis

46.

An odontoid fracture best amenable to anterior screw fixation is

A. Type I
B. Os odontoideum
C. Oblique downward from anterior to posterior
D. Associated with barrel chest
E. Malunited from trauma 9 months ago

47.

The approach with the *least* favorable outcome for thoracic disc herniation is

A. Laminectomy
B. Facetectomy
C. Transpedicular
D. Costotransversectomy
E. Lateral extracavitary

48.

The 10-year recurrence after microvascular decompression (MVD) for trigeminal neuralgia is

A. 10%
B. 20%
C. 30%
D. 50%
E. 80%

49.

The neurotransmitter from the locus ceruleus to the caudate nucleus is

A. Acetylcholine
B. Glutamate
C. Dopamine
D. Norepinephrine
E. Serotonin

50.

The two olfactory bulbs connect through

A. Fornix
B. Anterior commissure
C. Posterior commissure
D. Habenular commissure
E. None on the above

51.

All of the following tracts enter the cerebellum through the inferior cerebellar peduncle, *except*

A. Ventral spinocerebellar
B. Dorsal spinocerebellar
C. Ventral external arcuate fibers
D. Dorsal external arcuate fibers
E. Olivocerebellar

52.

What forms the posterior border of the anterior perforated substance?

A. Diagonal band of Broca
B. Medial longitudinal fasciculus
C. Stria medullaris
D. Stria terminalis
E. Indusium griseum

53.

Which nucleus of the oculomotor n carries general visceral efferent fibers?

A. Central nucleus
B. Medial nucleus
C. Lateral nucleus
D. Edinger–Westphal nucleus

54.

The trigeminal n supplies all of the following muscles, *except*

A. Masseter
B. Pterygoids
C. Tensor tympani
D. Anterior belly of digastric
E. Buccinator

55.

The general visceral efferent fibers of the glosso-pharyngeal nerve arise from the

A. Superior salivary nucleus
B. Inferior salivary nucleus
C. Rostral nucleus solitarius
D. Caudal nucleus solitarius
E. None of the above

56.

According to the head trauma guidelines, a patient with a brain contusion should have an intracranial pressure (ICP) monitor if his Glasgow Coma Scale (GCS) is

A. ≤8
B. ≤9
C. ≤10
D. ≤11
E. None of the above

57.

All of the following statements are true about the thalamic fasciculus, *except*

A. It is formed by the junction of the ansa lenticularis and lenticular fasciculus.
B. It carries information from the globus pallidus internus.
C. It relays information to the lateral posterior (LP) nucleus of thalamus.
D. It receives contribution from the contralateral deep cerebellar nuclei.
E. It uses GABA (gamma amino butyric acid) as a neurotransmitter.

58.

The stria terminalis connects

A. The hippocampus with the hypothalamus
B. The amygdala with the hypothalamus
C. The basal olfactory areas to the lateral hypothalamus
D. The midbrain to the hypothalamus
E. The hypothalamus to the anterior thalamic nucleus

59.

The main hippocampal direct cortical input is from the

A. Dentate gyrus
B. Alveus
C. Fimbria of fornix
D. Entorhinal cortex
E. Ammon's horn

60.

All of the following is true regarding the dentate nucleus of the cerebellum, *except*

A. It is part of the neocerebellum.
B. It projects to the contralateral thalamus.
C. Efferents pass through the superior cerebellar peduncle.
D. Output affects motor area 4.
E. It is supplied by PICA.

6   Answer Key 3

1.

D Putamen to globus pallidus externus

GABA and enkephalins are the main neurotransmitters from putamen to globus pallidus externus (GPe), GABA and substance P from GPe to globus pallidus internus (GPi), GABA from caudate to SN, GPe to STN, and GPi to thalamus. Ach is the main neurotransmitter from cerebral cortex to caudate, caudate to putamen, and lateral amygdala to cortex. Glutamate is the main neurotransmitter from cerebral cortex to putamen and STN, STN to GPe, GPi, and SN, thalamus to cortex and putamen. Dopamine is the main neurotransmitter from SN pars compacta to striatum, serotonin and cholecystokinin from dorsal raphe nucleus (DRN) to SN, serotonin and enkephalins from DRN to caudate (**Fig. 7**).

2.

C VLc (ventral lateral, pars caudalis) [Vop: ventralis oralis posterior and Vim: ventralis intermediate nucleus]

VL**c** (Vop and Vim) and VPLo receive input from dentate nucleus of the **c**erebellum and project to motor area 4, VA and VLo (Voa) receive input from GP and project to premotor cortex, MD from prefrontal cortex, temporal cortex, amygdala, SN, and GP and project to prefrontal cortex. LP receives input and projects to area 5 (**Fig. 8**).

3.

B Posteriorly

Basilar tip aneurysms pointing posteriorly carry the highest risk of perforator injury during clipping. Basilar tip aneurysms are now best treated endovascularly with coiling or stent-coiling.

4.

A Ulnar n

Wartenberg's sign consists of inability to adduct the little finger due to weakness of interossei secondary to ulnar n palsy. The little finger is abducted due to the unopposed action of extensor digiti minimi.

5.

C 4

1, Inferior sagittal sinus; 2, straight sinus; 3, internal cerebral v; 4, vein of Galen; 5, basal v of Rosenthal; 6, thalamostriate v; 7, transverse sinus; 8, superior sagittal sinus (**Fig. 5**).

6.

B 3

7.

B 2

1, Dentate gyrus; 2, Cornu Ammonis (hippocampus); 3, subiculum; 4, entorhinal cortex; 5, optic tract; 6, temporal horn of lateral ventricle; 7, fimbria of fornix; 8, tail of caudate nucleus; 9, alveus; 10, choroid plexus.

8.

A 1

9.

C Through 1

An endoscopic third ventriculostomy is done through the membrane (1) between the **M**ammillary bodies (2) and the **M**edian eminence; through the latter the pituitary infundibulum passes. The membrane (1) is part of the tuber cinereum (see also **Fig. 23B**).

10.

B 3

3, infundibular recess.

11.

A Glutamate

Glutamate is the main neurotransmitter from STN to GPe, GPi, and SN (**Fig. 7**).

12.

A Prefrontal cortex

MD from prefrontal cortex, temporal cortex, amygdala, SN, and GP and project to prefrontal cortex (**Fig. 8**).

13.

A 1

In this endoscopic view of the right lateral ventricle, the fornix (1) forms the superior and anterior boundary of the foramen of Monro (4). The choroid plexus is observed between the septum pellucidum (3) and thalamus (2).

14.

D Posterior part of the posterior limb

The corticospinal fibers occupy the posterior half of the posterior limb of the internal capsule with the legs represented posteriorly, corticobulbar the genu, auditory projections in sublenticular (inferior thalamic peduncle), visual in retrolenticular (posterior thalamic peduncle). The anterior limb contains the anterior thalamic peduncle, while the posterior limb contains the superior thalamic peduncle (**Fig. 6**).

15.

E Granule cells

Excitatory structures in the cerebellum include: climbing fibers, mossy fibers, and granule cells. All other cells are inhibitory (**Fig. 11**).

16.

D 26%

Based on NASCET, carotid endarterectomy reduces the risk of stroke from 26% to 9% over 2 years in symptomatic patients with 70–99% stenosis.

Further Reading: North American Symptomatic Carotid Endarterectomy Trial Collaborators. Beneficial effect of carotid endarterectomy in symptomatic patients with high-grade carotid stenosis. *N Engl J Med.* 1991;325:445–453

17.

B 1–2%

The annual risk of rupture of cavernomas is 0.5–1%, aneurysms 1–2%, AVMs 2–4%. After AVM rupture: mortality 10%, morbidity 30%, rebleed 6% in the first 6 months. After aneurysm rupture, prehospital death is 50%, of the remaining patients there is 20% mortality, 20% morbidity, rebleed 50% in 6 months worst in the first 24 hours.

18.

B Cavernous

The cavernous carotid a gives the McConnell's capsular a, the inferior cavernous a, and the meningohypophyseal trunk. The meningohypophyseal trunk gives the dorsal meningeal a, inferior hypophyseal a, and the tentorial artery of Bernasconi and Cassinari. The petrous carotid gives off vidian, caroticotympanic, and occasionally stapedial aa. The ophthalmic segment: ophthalmic and superior hypophyseal aa, the communicating segment: posterior communicating and anterior choroidal aa.

19.

C 50 mL/100 g/min

The normal cerebral blood flow is 50 mL/100 g/min, with higher flow in the gray matter than the white matter. In the ischemic penumbra, it is 8–23 mL/100 g/min. The normal Oxygen consumption is 3.5 mL/100 g/min.

20.

D Area postrema

The circumventricular organs are devoid of BBB except the subcommissural organ. The subfornical organ and organum vasculosum detect serum osmolarity. The area postrema is the only paired organ and it induces emesis (**Fig. 24B**).

21.

C 450 mL/d

The normal adult CSF volume is 150 mL, of which 30 mL intraventricular, 40 mL spinal subarachnoid space, and 80 mL cranial subarachnoid space. The body produces 3 times the CSF volume per day (450 mL).

22.

D Ophthalmic

Branches of the ophthalmic segment of ICA: ophthalmic and superior hypophyseal aa.

23.

E None of the above

The anterior choroidal a is a branch of the communicating segment of the ICA, has cisternal and plexal segments, and supplies internal capsule, optic chiasm, optic tract, optic radiation, thalamus, GP, cerebral peduncle, SN, red nucleus, and choroid plexus of lateral ventricle.

24.

A Percheron

The a of Percheron is a variant unpaired branch of the PCA supplying thalamus and midbrain bilaterally. Occlusion causes bilateral thalamic infarcts.

25.

E The cervical carotid a to the vertebral a

The proatlantal a is an anastomosis between the vertebral artery and either the ICA or ECA; it travels between the occiput and C1. The hypoglossal a (0.1%) connects the ICA to the basilar a and travels through the hypoglossal canal. The acoustic (otic) a connects the ICA to the basilar a through the internal auditory canal. The primitive trigeminal a (0.5%) connects ICA to basilar a.

26.

E Layer V

In a 6-layer cortex model of Lorente de No, the main output from the internal pyramidal layer (V) is to the brain stem and spinal cord, from the multiform layer (VI) to the thalamus. The main afferents connect to the internal granular layer (IV). The molecular (I), external granular (II), and external pyramidal (III) layers connect to other cortical areas, while III connects the 2 hemispheres.

27.

A Orbital frontal gyri to anterior temporal lobe

The uncinate fasciculus connects orbito-frontal gyri to anterior temporal lobe. The arcuate fasciculus connects the superior and middle frontal gyri to the temporal lobe. The superior longitudinal fasciculus: frontal to parietal and occipital. The inferior longitudinal fasciculus: temporal to occipital.

28.

D Parietal cortex

The corticospinal tract originates from parietal cortex (40%), premotor (30%), and motor (30%). Only 3% of fibers arise from Betz cells.

29.

B Vim (ventralis intermediate)

DBS for tremors (essential or Parkinsonian) targets Vim; bradykinesia and rigidity (Parkinson) targets STN; dystonia targets GPi.

30.

A Dopamine

Dopamine is the main neurotransmitter from SN pars compacta to striatum, serotonin and cholecystokinin from dorsal raphe nucleus (DRN) to SN, serotonin and enkephalins from DRN to caudate. GABA and enkephalins are the main neurotransmitters from putamen to GPe, GABA and substance P from GPe to GPi and from putamen to GPi, GABA from caudate to SN, GPe to STN, and GPi to thalamus. Ach is the main neurotransmitter from cerebral cortex to caudate, caudate to putamen, and lateral amygdala to cortex. Glutamate is the main neurotransmitter from cerebral cortex to putamen and STN, STN to GPe, GPi, and SN, thalamus to cortex and putamen (**Fig. 7**).

31.

D 50%

Rebleeding from intracranial aneurysm is 20% in 2 weeks, 50% in 6 months. This is highest in the first 24 hours, especially the first 6 hours after subarachnoid hemorrhage.

32.

C 3

The main features of the Hunt and Hess grading system for subarachnoid hemorrhage: grade 1: no or mild headache; 2: moderate-to-severe headache or cranial nerve deficits; 3: lethargy, confusion; 4: hemiparesis, stupor; 5: extensor posturing, coma (**Table 22**).

33.

B 7%

The presented AVM is Spetzler–Martin grade 4 (**Table 20**), surgical morbidity: minor deficit 20%, major deficit 7%. Grade 5, minor deficit 19%, major deficit 12%. Grade 3, minor deficit 12%, major deficit 4%.

34.

E Surgical evacuation

Subdural empyema is a surgical emergency due to the risk of venous thrombosis and cerebral infarct.

35.

E Zygoma

The pterion is H-shaped and is made of: frontal, parietal, squamous part of temporal bone, and the greater wing of the sphenoid bone.

36.

D They synapse in the caudal part of the nucleus of tractus solitarius.

The nucleus of tractus solitarius cranial part connects to the facial n, middle part glossopharyngeal n, caudal part vagus n (**Fig. 14**).

37.

A Adductor pollicis

Adductor pollicis is supplied by the ulnar n. The remaining muscles (LOAF) are supplied by the median n.

38.

B Superior oblique

The superior oblique is supplied by the trochlear n, the lateral rectus abducens n, the remaining muscles oculomotor n.

39.

C Trochlear n

Structures entering the orbit outside the annulus of Zinn are: LFT: Lacrimal n (from V_1), Frontal n (from V_1), Trochlear n (IV), in addition to the superior ophthalmic vein.

40.

C Facial and superior vestibular

In the internal acoustic meatus, the facial n is above the cochlear n (7-up, coke down), the superior vestibular n is above the inferior vestibular n, and the facial n is medial to the superior vestibular n and separated from it by the Bill's bar (**Fig. 14**).

41.

D Membrana tectoria

The membrana tectoria is the cranial extension of the PLL and connects C2 to clivus. The transverse ligament of atlas is anterior to it. There is another tectorial membrane in the inner ear and is involved with hearing.

42.

B Lateral spinothalamic

The lateral (neo) spinothalamic tract transmits pain and temperature from the contralateral body and is somatotopically organized with the legs laterally. The ventral (paleo) spinothalamic is involved in light touch. The gracil and cuneate tracts carry fine touch and proprioception from lower and upper halves of the body, respectively (**Fig. 15**).

43.

A II

Substance P is the main neurotransmitter in the substantia gelatinosa of Rolando (II) and is involved in pain sensation.

44.

C Ulnar n

The arcade of Struthers when present stretches between the medial head of triceps and medial intermuscular septum and can be associated with ulnar n compression above the elbow, while the ligaMent of Struthers is associated with Median n entrapment.

45.

E Adductor pollicis

Froment's test is performed by asking the patient to hold a piece of paper between the thumb and index fingers. In case of ulnar palsy, the patient loses adductor pollicis. As the examiner tries to pull the paper, the patient compensates by flexing the distal phalanx of the thumb using flexor pollicis longus supplied by the AIN (a branch of the median n).

46.

C Oblique downward from anterior to posterior

Typical indication for an anterior odontoid screw is type II fracture, when the fracture line is horizontal or oblique downward from anterior to posterior. Barrel chest is a contraindication. Malunion is a relative contraindication unless decortication of the fracture surface is performed. Type I and III are usually treated in a collar. Os odontoideum is typically treated by posterior C1–C2 fusion.

Further Reading: Ryken TC, Hadley MN, Aarabi B, et al. Management of isolated fractures of the axis in adults. *Neurosurgery* 2013 Mar;72(Suppl 2):132–150

47.

A Laminectomy

Thoracic disc herniation can be successfully treated by a transpedicular, transfacet, costotransversectomy, extracavitary, or transthoracic (open or endoscopic) approaches. Laminectomy has a high risk of worsening motor function.

48.

C 30%

Recurrence after MVD for trigeminal neuralgia is 15% at 5 years and 30% at 10 years, glycerol rhizotomy 54% at 4 years, and SRS 20% at 3 years.

49.

D Norepinephrine

NE is the main neurotransmitter output from locus ceruleus and is involved in REM sleep (**Figs. 7 and 31**).

50.

B Anterior commissure

Fibers from the medial olfactory stria cross to the contralateral side through the anterior commissure.

51.

A Ventral spinocerebellar

The ventral spinocerebellar tract enters the cerebellum through the superior cerebellar peduncle. It is predominantly contralateral and originates in the lower extremities (**Fig. 11**).

52.

A Diagonal band of Broca

The diagonal band of Broca forms the posterior border of the anterior perforated substance.

53.

D Edinger–Westphal nucleus

Edinger–Westphal nucleus provides parasympathetic component of the oculomotor n (III) (general visceral efferent). The general somatic efferents arise from the central nucleus supplying levator palpebrae superioris bilaterally, medial nucleus supplying contralateral superior rectus, and lateral nucleus supplying ipsilateral inferior rectus, inferior oblique and medial rectus (**Fig. 14**).

54.

E Buccinator

The facial n supplies the buccinator (buccal n).

55.

B Inferior salivary nucleus

The general visceral efferents of the glossopharyngeal n originate in the inferior salivary nucleus, travel through the lesser petrosal n, synapse in the otic ganglion, then supply the parotid gland through the auriculotemporal n (**Fig. 14**).

56.

A £8

Based on the brain trauma foundation guidelines, ICP monitoring should be placed in cases of:

a. GCS ≤8 and a positive head CT.
b. GCS ≤8, a negative head CT, and 2 of the following:
   i. Age >40
   ii. SBP <90
   iii. Posturing

Further Reading: The Brain Trauma Foundation. The American Association of Neurological Surgeons. The Joint Section on Neurotrauma and Critical Care. Indications for intracranial pressure monitoring. *J Neurotrauma* 2000 Jun-Jul;17(6-7):479–491

57.

C It relays information to the lateral posterior (LP) nucleus of thalamus.

The LP nucleus of thalamus receives input from area 5 and projects to areas 5 and 7 (**Figs. 7 and 8**).

58.

B The amygdala with the hypothalamus

The stria terminalis connects amygdala to hypothalamus and septal nuclei (**Fig. 9**).

59.

D Entorhinal cortex

The main cortical input to hippocampus is from entorhinal cortex, through the alvear (to CA1) or perforant (to dentate gyrus and CA3) pathways (**Fig. 4**).

Further Reading: Amaral DG. Emerging principles of intrinsic hippocampal organization. *Curr Opin Neurobiol.* 1993 Apr;3(2):225–229

60.

E It is supplied by PICA.

The blood supply of the dentate nucleus is from the superior cerebellar a (**Fig. 11**).

7 Test 4—Pathology and Radiology

1.

The anterior neuropore closes at which gestational age?

A. 13 days
B. 17 days
C. 22 days
D. 24 days
E. 28 days

2.

The following histologic finding is characteristic of

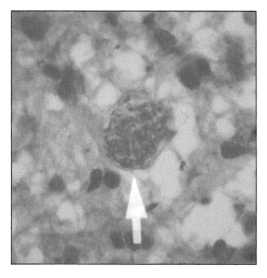

A. Glioblastoma multiformes
B. Toxoplasmosis
C. Subependymal giant cell astrocytoma
D. Bacterial brain abscess
E. Cysticercosis

3.

Which disease is X-linked recessive, characterized by ceramide accumulation in the tissues, and manifests as corneal opacities, cerebrovascular occlusions, peripheral neuropathy, and skin angiokeratomas?

A. Fabry's disease
B. Niemann–Pick's disease
C. Tay–Sachs disease
D. Hurler's disease
E. Gaucher's disease

4.

The abnormality depicted in the following MRI is caused by

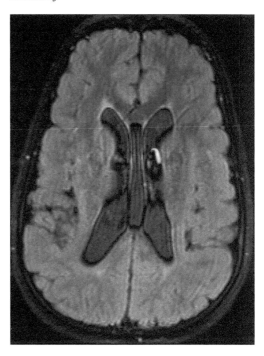

A. Primary neurulation defect
B. Abnormal disjunction
C. Abnormal ventral induction
D. Abnormal migration

5.

All of the following are characteristics of Wilson's disease, *except*

A. Kayser–Fleischer ring of the cornea
B. Liver cirrhosis
C. Spongiform red degeneration of the lentiform nucleus
D. Opalski cells
E. Increase serum copper (Cu)

6.

The following tumor was removed from the frontal lobe of a 35-year-old male with seizures. What is the diagnosis?

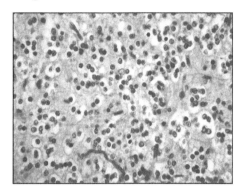

A. Central neurocytoma
B. Fibrillary astrocytoma
C. Oligodendroglioma
D. Ganglioglioma
E. Dysembryoplastic neuroepithelial tumor (DNET)

7.

The mechanism that best describes the following CT finding is

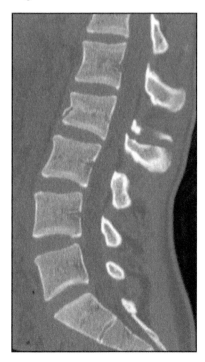

A. Axial load
B. Extension injury
C. Flexion injury
D. Distraction injury
E. Flexion and distraction injury

8.

The following neural tube defect occurs at which gestational age?

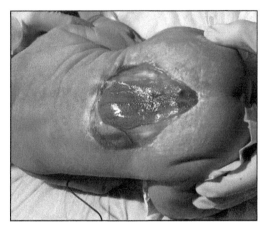

A. 3–4 weeks
B. 4–5 weeks
C. 5–10 weeks
D. 2–5 months
E. 6–7 months

9.

Which disease is autosomal recessive characterized by Zebra bodies, gargoyle face, thick meninges, and hepatosplenomegaly?

A. Morquio's syndrome
B. Krabbe's disease
C. Maroteaux–Lamy syndrome
D. Hurler's disease
E. Sly's syndrome

10.

Refsum's disease is characterized by all of the following, *except*

A. Autosomal recessive
B. Cu/Zn superoxide dismutase deficiency
C. Peripheral neuropathy
D. Retinitis pigmentosum
E. Cardiomyopathy

11.

Which vasculopathy is characterized by orogenital ulcers, uveitis, ulcerative colitis, and meningo-encephalitis?

A. Behçet's disease
B. Takayasu's arteritis
C. Kawasaki's disease
D. Wegener's granulomatosis
E. Polyarteritis nodosa

12.

Gorlin's syndrome, which includes medulloblastoma, meningioma, and basal cell nevus syndrome is caused by an abnormality of which chromosome?

A. 3
B. 5
C. 9
D. 10
E. 17

13.

The following brain tumor is seen in which disease?

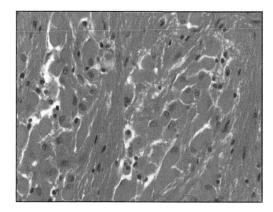

A. Von Hippel–Lindau disease
B. Tuberous sclerosis
C. Neurofibromatosis 1
D. Neurofibromatosis 2
E. Li–Fraumeni syndrome

14.

Which of the following is *not* a mitochondrial myopathy?

A. MELAS (myopathy, encephalopathy, lactic acidosis, and stroke-like episodes)
B. MERRF (myoclonic epilepsy with ragged red fibers)
C. MNGIE (mitochondrial neurogastrointestinal encephalopathy)
D. Kearns–Sayre syndrome
E. Familial periodic paralysis

15.

Neurofibrillary tangles and neuritic plaques are found in which disease?

A. Alzheimer's disease
B. Pick's disease
C. Huntington's chorea
D. Parkinson's disease
E. Shy-Drager disease

16.

The following tissue is from a temporal lobe lesion of a child with seizures. What is the diagnosis?

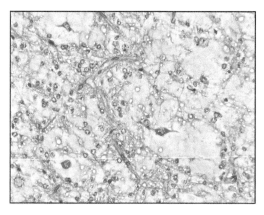

A. Ganglioglioma
B. Dysembryoplastic neuroepithelial tumor (DNET)
C. Chondrosarcoma
D. Oligodendroglioma
E. Central neurocytoma

17.

The congenital abnormality in the following MRI is caused by

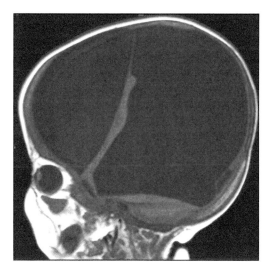

A. Primary neurulation defect
B. Abnormal disjunction
C. Abnormal ventral induction
D. Abnormal migration

18.

Which type of headache is unilateral, more common in males, associated with rhinorrhea, lacrimation, and conjunctival injection?

A. Classic migraine
B. Common migraine
C. Cluster headache
D. Trigeminal neuralgia
E. Ramsay Hunt syndrome

19.

The tumor depicted below was recovered from the cerebellum of a patient with abnormality of which chromosome?

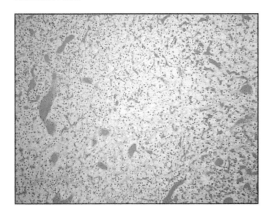

A. 3
B. 5
C. 9
D. 17
E. 22

20.

Which toxicity is characterized by encephalitis, peripheral neuropathy, and basophilic stippling of red blood corpuscles?

A. Mercury
B. Methotrexate
C. Arsenic
D. Manganese
E. Lead

21.

The finding in the following MRI is suggestive of

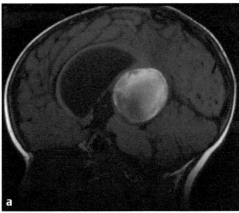

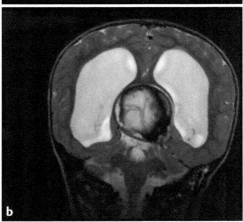

A. Germinoma
B. Tectal glioma
C. Pineal teratoma
D. Vein of Galen malformation
E. Giant aneurysm of the posterior cerebral artery (PCA)

22.
Based on the following CT scan, what is the most important next step in the management of this patient?

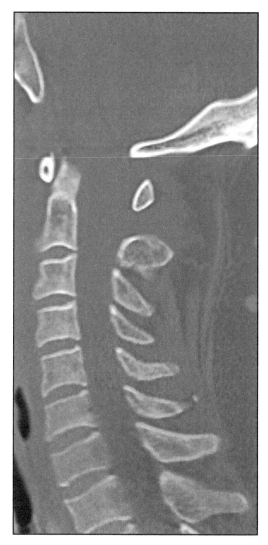

A. Gardners–Wells traction
B. Halo-vest
C. Posterior C1–C2 fusion
D. Anterior odontoid screw
E. None of the above, this is a normal finding

23.
The following tissue was removed from a C2 vertebral body lesion. What is the diagnosis?

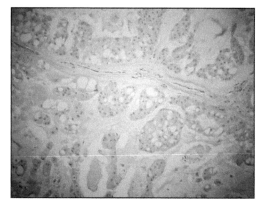

A. Chondrosarcoma
B. Chordoma
C. Metastatic carcinoma
D. Osteoid osteoma
E. Osseous meningioma

24.
Which leukodystrophy is X-linked recessive characterized by tigroid pattern on the MRI, mental retardation, ataxia, nystagmus, and spasticity?

A. Krabbe's disease
B. Metachromatic leukodystrophy
C. Pelizaeus–Merzbacher disease
D. Canavan's disease
E. Alexander's disease

25.
All of the following side-effects can be observed with carbamazepine, *except*

A. Hypernatremia
B. Teratogenicity
C. Toxic hepatitis
D. Pancytopenia
E. Ataxia

26.

The following tissue was removed from the brain of a child with seizures, what is the most likely diagnosis?

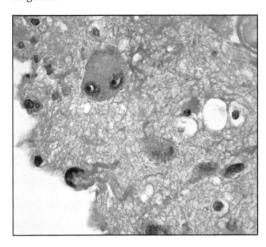

A.   Ganglioglioma
B.   Dysembryoplastic neuroepithelial tumor (DNET)
C.   Subependymal giant cell astrocytoma (SEGA)
D.   Oligodendroglioma
E.   Central neurocytoma

27.

The finding on the following CTA is suggestive of

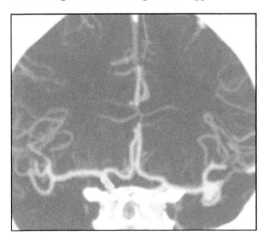

A.   ACOM aneurysm
B.   Right ophthalmic artery aneurysm
C.   Left ophthalmic artery aneurysm
D.   Right MCA aneurysm
E.   Left MCA aneurysm

28.

Amyotrophic lateral sclerosis is featured by abnormalities of

A.   Dystrophin
B.   Acid maltase
C.   Ryanodine
D.   Mitochondria
E.   Cu/Zn superoxide dismutase

29.

Tolosa–Hunt syndrome includes all of the following, *except*

A.   Painless
B.   Ophthalmoplegia
C.   Sensory loss over the forehead
D.   Superior orbital fissure inflammation
E.   Treated with steroids

30.

Which disease is X-linked recessive characterized by decreased copper absorption, diffuse neuronal loss, mental retardation, seizures, and intracranial aneurysms?

A.   Lesch–Nyhan disease
B.   Menke's kinky hair disease
C.   Wilson's disease
D.   Lowe's syndrome
E.   Leber's disease

31.

The tumor depicted below typically has all of the following radiological characteristics, *except*

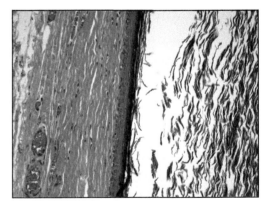

A.   Cerebellopontine angle location
B.   Hypodense on CT
C.   Hypointense on T1-weighted MRI
D.   Hyperintense on T2-weighted MRI
E.   No restricted diffusion

32.

The following histology represents a lesion removed from the skull of a child. What is the diagnosis?

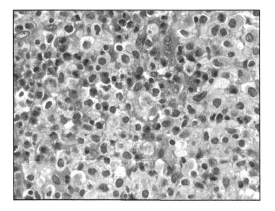

A. Lymphoma
B. Metastatic carcinoma
C. Chordoma
D. Eosinophilic granuloma
E. Cysticercosis

33.

The following imaging finding is characteristic of

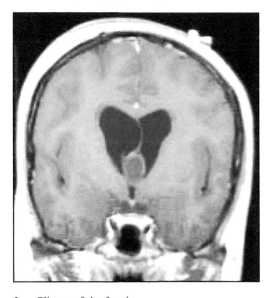

A. Glioma of the fornix
B. Subependymoma
C. Colloid cyst
D. Subependymal giant cell astrocytoma (SEGA)
E. Rathke's cleft cyst

34.

A cherry-red spot in the macula is observed in all of the following diseases, *except*

A. GM1 gangliosidosis
B. Sandhoff's disease
C. Tay–Sachs disease
D. Gaucher's disease
E. Niemann–Pick disease

35.

Which X-linked recessive disease is characterized by atrophy of the shoulder and pelvic girdles, calf pseudohypertrophy, and congestive heart failure?

A. Duchenne's muscle dystrophy
B. Emery–Dreifuss syndrome
C. Facioscapulohumeral muscle dystrophy
D. Oculopharyngeal muscle dystrophy
E. McArdle's disease

36.

The presence of Negri bodies in the hippocampus and cerebellum is characteristic of

A. Measles
B. Rabies
C. Amyotrophic lateral sclerosis (ALS)
D. Alzheimer's disease
E. Parkinson's disease

37.

All of the following features are true about the tumor depicted below, *except*

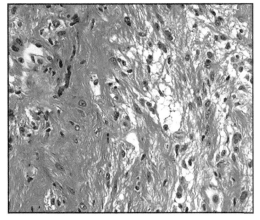

A. Commonly occurs in children
B. Frequently in the posterior fossa
C. Rarely cystic
D. Complete surgical resection is curative
E. Prognosis is good

38.
Macrocephaly is observed with which metabolic disease?

A. Phenylketonuria
B. Gaucher's disease
C. Krabbe's disease
D. Pelizaeus–Merzbacher disease
E. Canavan's disease

39.
The abnormality depicted by the following angiogram is located at the

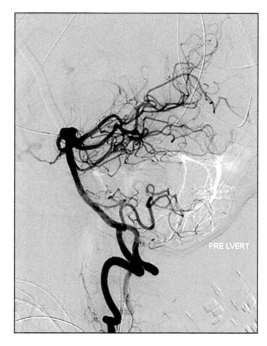

A. Vertebrobasilar junction
B. Posterior inferior cerebellar artery (PICA)
C. Anterior inferior cerebellar artery (AICA)
D. Superior cerebellar artery (SCA)
E. Basilar tip

40.
Intracytoplasmic Bunina bodies can be found in

A. Measles
B. Rabies
C. Amyotrophic lateral sclerosis (ALS)
D. Alzheimer's disease
E. Parkinson's disease

41.
The following histological picture is observed with which disease?

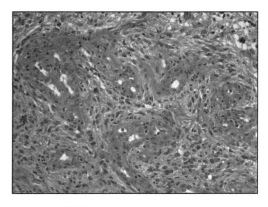

A. Medulloblastoma
B. Ependymoma
C. Glioblastoma multiforme (GBM)
D. Meningioma
E. Gemistocytic astrocytoma

42.
All of the following is true about the one-and-a-half syndrome, *except*

A. One eye can't abduct or adduct
B. The other eye can't abduct
C. There is bilateral medial longitudinal fasciculus (MLF) injury
D. Common cause is ischemia
E. Could be caused by demyelination (multiple sclerosis)

43.
The best treatment for drop attacks is

A. Temporal lobectomy
B. Vagal nerve stimulator
C. Hemispherectomy
D. Corpus callosotomy
E. Multiple subpial transections

44.

The aneurysm depicted in the following angiogram is located at

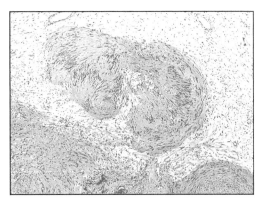

A. PCOM (posterior communicating artery)
B. ACOM (anterior communicating artery)
C. Cavernous carotid artery
D. Carotid terminus
E. MCA (middle cerebral artery)

45.

A 35-year-old female has decreased vision and the following flair MRI. What is the most likely diagnosis?

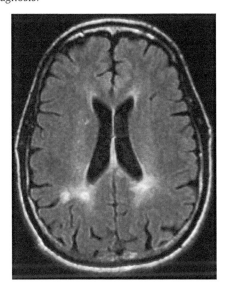

A. Pseudotumor cerebri
B. Multiple sclerosis (MS)
C. Brain abscesses
D. Lymphoma
E. Multifocal glioblastoma multiforme

46.

The following tumor is found in patients with abnormalities in which chromosome?

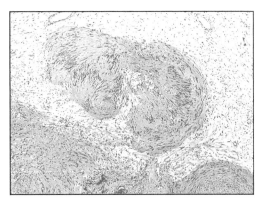

A. 3
B. 5
C. 10
D. 17
E. 22

47.

What is the abnormality in the following axial T2-weighted MRI at L4–L5?

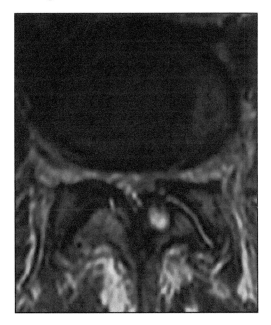

A. An extruded disc fragment
B. An arachnoid cyst
C. A synovial cyst
D. A schwannoma
E. A meningioma

48.
The following histology is found in

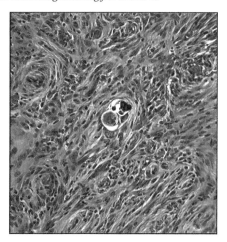

A. Meningioma
B. Glioblastoma multiforme
C. Medulloblastoma
D. Ganglioglioma
E. Neurofibroma

49.
A 52-year-old female presents with quadriparesis and tingling. Based on the following MRI, what is the most likely diagnosis?

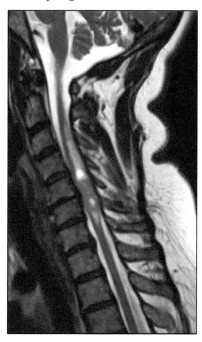

A. Ependymoma
B. Astrocytoma
C. Hemangioblastoma
D. Syringomyelia
E. Transverse myelitis

50.
All of the following is true about spinal dural arteriovenous fistulae (type I), *except*

A. Usually acquired
B. Age range 40–70 years old
C. Low flow
D. Low pressure
E. Present with venous hypertension

51.
Oculopalatal myoclonus is caused by an injury of

A. Medial longitudinal fasciculus
B. Guillain–Mollaret triangle
C. Substantia nigra
D. Fastigial nucleus
E. Nucleus accumbens septi

52.
Lambert–Eaton myasthenic syndrome (LEMS) is caused by which antibodies?

A. Anti-Hu
B. Anti-Tr
C. Anti-Ri
D. Anti-AchR (acetylcholine receptor)
E. Anti-VGCC (voltage-gated calcium channel)

53.
Benedikt's syndrome is caused by a lesion of

A. Cranial nerve IV
B. Cranial nerve VI
C. Cranial nerve IX
D. Red nucleus
E. Substantia nigra

54.
When the following tumor occurs in the tectum, what is the best treatment?

A. Conventional radiation
B. Stereotactic radiosurgery
C. Chemotherapy
D. Gross total resection
E. Shunt for hydrocephalus

55.
The histology of the tumor depicted below most likely will show all of the following, *except*

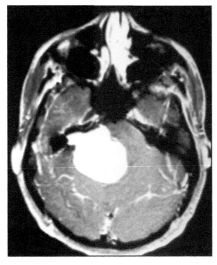

A. Antoni A
B. Antoni B
C. School of fish
D. Keratin
E. Verocay bodies

56.
The following CT shows

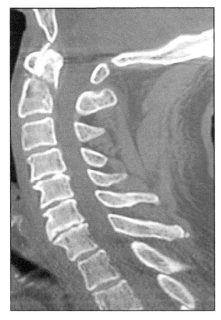

A. Os odontoideum
B. Type I dens fracture
C. Type II dens fracture
D. Type III dens fracture
E. Type IV dens fracture

57.
What structure is depicted in the following figure?

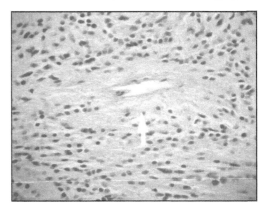

A. Pseudorosette
B. Pseudopalisading necrosis
C. Verocay body
D. Homer–Wright rosette
E. Flexner–Wintersteiner rosette

58.
Canavan's disease is characterized by all of the following, *except*

A. Autosomal recessive
B. Blindness
C. Mental retardation
D. Macrocephaly
E. Arylsulfatase A deficiency

59.
Malignant hyperthermia is associated with which abnormality?

A. Porphobilinogen deaminase
B. Ryanodine receptor
C. Mitochondrial DNA
D. Phytanic acid oxidase
E. Cu/Zn superoxide dismutase

60.
Gaucher's disease is associated with all of the following, *except*

A. Autosomal recessive
B. Glucocerebrosidase deficiency
C. Macrocephaly
D. Hepatosplenomegaly
E. Wrinkled tissue-paper appearing cells

8 Answer Key 4

1.

D 24 days

The neural tube closure starts in the middle at 22 days, then the anterior neuropore at 24 days forming the lamina terminalis, and then the posterior neuropore at 28 days.

2.

B Toxoplasmosis

*B*radyzoites are *b*ound in a cyst (*b*ag) while tachyzoites are loose. They are both characteristic of toxoplasmosis. The infection risk is higher in AIDS patients. The lesions are ring enhancing and appear as a target sign on CT or MRI.

3.

A Fabry's disease

Fabry's disease is a lysosomal storage disease, X-lin*k*ed re*c*essive, characterized by α-gala*c*tosidase A deficiency. It causes *c*eramide (sphingosine + long-chain fatty acid) a*cc*umulation in tissues, *c*orneal opacities, *c*erebrovascular o*cc*lusions, *C*AD, *k*idney insufficiency, s*k*in angio*k*eratomas, and wea*k*ness from peripheral neuropathy (**Table 12**).

4.

D Abnormal migration

Cavum vergae and polymicrogyria are both caused by abnormal migration and occur at 2–5 months gestation (**Table 9**).

5.

E Increase serum copper (Cu)

In Wilson's disease, there is decreased serum Cu and ceruloplasmin, increased urinary Cu (**Table 14**).

6.

C Oligodendroglioma

Oligodendrogliomas are characterized by small round nuclei and clear cytoplasm (perinuclear halo, artifact) giving it fried egg-yolk or bee-hive appearance. They also have chicken-wire vascular pattern. The presence of 1p19q deletion is a good prognostic factor. It favors response to chemotherapy: PCV (Procarbazine, CCNU [lomustine], Vincristine) or temozolomide. In the absence of increased cellularity, mitotic figures, cellular pleomorphism, and endothelial proliferation, the tumor shown is WHO grade II. Patients with WHO grade III (anaplastic oligodendroglioma) should get radiotherapy as well.

7.

E Flexion and distraction injury

The typical mechanism for a Chance fracture is a seat-belt injury with flexion distraction.

8.

A 3–4 weeks

Myelomeningocele is a disorder of primary neurulation that occurs at 3–4 weeks gestation (**Table 9**). Surgery (closure) should be performed within 48 hours of birth to avoid meningitis and in some specialized centers intrauterine (prenatal, fetal) surgery is done. The brain should be screened for hydrocephalus. With fetal surgery, there is less need for shunting and better functional outcome, but more premature delivery and uterine dehiscence.

9.

D Hurler's disease

These are features of Hurler's disease, which is a mucopolysaccharidose (MPS IH). It is caused by α-L-iduronidase deficiency and urine shows increased dermatan sulfate (**Table 12**).

10.

B Cu/Zn superoxide dismutase deficiency

Refsum's disease is caused by phytanic acid oxidase deficiency. Cu/Zn superoxide dismutase deficiency is a feature of ALS (**Table 13**).

11.

A Behçet's disease

Behçet's disease is characterized by orogenital ulcers, uveitis, ulcerative colitis, meningoencephalitis, brain stem edema, confusion, erythema nodosum, and polyarthritis (**Table 29**). Treatment includes corticosteroids.

12.

C 9

Gorlin's syndrome is inherited as autosomal dominant on chromosome 9 (**Table 11**).

13.

B Tuberous sclerosis

Large astrocytes with large eccentric nuclei are characteristics of SEGA. SEGA occurs in 15% of patients with tuberous sclerosis. Tuberous sclerosis is inherited as autosomal dominant on chromosome 9 or 16 (**Table 11**).

14.

E Familial periodic paralysis

Mitochondrial myopathies inherited through maternal mitochondria include MELAS, MERRF, MNGIE, Luft's, and Leigh's diseases. Kearns–Sayre is a defect in mitochondrial DNA not maternally inherited. Familial periodic paralysis is caused by a genetic defect coding for Ca in muscle fiber membranes (**Table 13**).

15.

A Alzheimer's disease

Alzheimer's disease is characterized by neurofibrillary tangles (tau protein), neuritic plaques (beta amyloid), Hirano bodies, and lack of cholinergic output from the amygdala to the cerebral cortex (**Tables 10 and 14, Fig. 7**). Treatment includes donepezil (Aricept) which is an acetylcholinesterase inhibitor.

16.

B Dysembryoplastic neuroepithelial tumor (DNET)

In DNET neurons are floating in mucinous material, small cells resemble oligodendrocytes, and vessels have a chicken-wire pattern.

17.

C Abnormal ventral induction

Alobar holoprosencephaly occurs at 5–10 weeks gestation and is caused by abnormal ventral induction (**Table 9**).

18.

C Cluster headache

Cluster headache is characterized by increased parasympathetic discharge causing hypersecretions. Classic migraine has aura while common migraine has no aura. Tolosa–Hunt is painful ophthalmoplegia and Ramsay Hunt is herpes zoster of the geniculate ganglion.

19.

A 3

Clear cells (lipid content) occur in hemangioblastoma. They stain positive for vimentin while renal cell carcinoma stain positive for EMA and cytokeratin. When part of von Hippel–Lindau disease, it is inherited as autosomal dominant on chromosome 3 (**Table 11**).

20.

E Lead

Basophilic stippling of RBCs is found in cases of lead poisoning, Mees' lines (white on finger nails) in arsenic cases, cerebellar tremors and renal tubular necrosis in mercury poisoning, parkinsonism in manganese toxicity, and subacute necrotizing leukoencephalitis (SNLE) with methotrexate (**Table 30**).

21.

D Vein of Galen malformation

A well-circumscribed mass in the pineal region with various MRI signal from blood products is consistent with a diagnosis of Vein of Galen malformation. In neonates, high cardiac output heart failure can be fatal and may warrant urgent treatment, preferably endovascular. In older children, it can cause obstructive hydrocephalus.

22.

B Halo-vest

Atlanto-occipital dislocation is evidenced by increase in the basion-dens interval. CTA or MRA would be important to rule out associated vascular injuries. Halo-vest stabilization with some axial compression is an important next step. Definitive treatment will require posterior occipito-cervical fusion. C1–C2 fusion will not fix the instability which is between C1 and the occiput. Traction would be detrimental. The odontoid is intact.

23.

B Chordoma

Chordomas are characterized by physaliphorous cells and a mucinous background. They are common in the sacrum and clivus and have a bright T2 signal on MRI. The best cure is en-bloc resection. Proton-beam radiation could be helpful if there is residual tumor.

24.

C Pelizaeus–Merzbacher disease

Pelizaeus–Merzbacher disease is an X-linked recessive leukodystrophy caused by a defect in synthesis of proteolipid lipoprotein. It causes mental retardation with cerebellar involvement, ataxia, nystagmus, spasticity, and tigroid pattern on MRI (**Table 12**).

25.

A Hypernatremia

Carbamazepine causes hyponatremia (**Table 34**). The mechanism is SIADH. Treatment includes water restriction and discontinuing the drug. Other anti-epileptics causing hyponatremia: lamotrigine, oxcarbazepine, and valproate.

26.

A Ganglioglioma

Large multinucleated ganglion cells are present in ganglioglioma. Perivascular lymphocytes can also be observed. These tumors as well as DNET are common in children and cause seizures.

27.

E Left MCA aneurysm

Left MCA aneurysm (*arrow*) is observed on the following brain CTA.

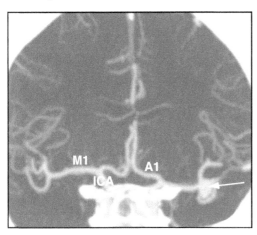

28.

E Cu/Zn superoxide dismutase

ALS is associated with Cu/Zn superoxide dismutase mutation. Ryanodine receptor mutation is seen in malignant hyperthermia. Dystrophin anomalies are present in musclular dystrophies (Duchenne, Becker, and limb–girdle). Acid maltase deficiency is a feature of Pompe's disease. Maternal mitochondrial abnormalities include MELAS, MERRF, MNGIE, Luft's, and Leigh's diseases (**Table 13**).

29.

A Painless

Tolosa–Hunt syndrome is a painful ophthalmoplegia (**Table 15**).

30.

B Menke's kinky hair disease

Menke's kinky hair disease is X-linked recessive and is characterized by decreased cupper absorption, mental retardation, colorless brittle hair, and tortuous abdominal viscera (**Table 12**). Wilson's disease is autosomal recessive (chromosome 13) and is characterized by Cu deposition in the lentiform nucleus and liver, *Kayser–Fleischer* ring in cornea, decreased total serum Cu and ceruloplasmin, increased urinary Cu. However, free (unbound) serum Cu can be elevated (**Table 14**).

31.

E No restricted diffusion

Epidermoid cyst is evident by stratified squamous epithelium and abundant keratin with no hair follicles. There is typically restricted diffusion on MRI. Dermoid cysts have hair follicles in addition.

32.

D Eosinophilic granuloma

Bilobed nuclei of eosinophils (*black arrowhead*), foamy macrophages (*white arrow*), and large grooved nuclei (*black arrow*) are seen in eosinophilic granuloma (Langerhans cell histiocytosis).

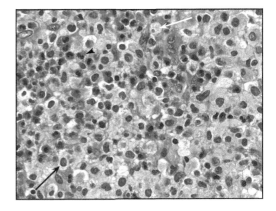

33.

C Colloid cyst

Colloid cysts of the third ventricle occur in the region of the foramen of Monro and cause obstructive hydrocephalus. They are typically hyperdense on CT. On MRI, they are hyperintense on T1, hypointense on T2, but the reverse could occur depending on the cyst content. Histologically they are lined by a single layer of columnar cells.

34.

D Gaucher's disease

Lysosomal storage diseases (sphingolipidoses) are typically characterized by a cherry-red spot in the macula except for Gaucher's disease and Fabry's disease (**Table 12**).

35.

A Duchenne's muscle dystrophy

Duchenne's muscle dystrophy is caused by decreased dystrophin. Patients have a positive Gower's test, respiratory infections, increased CK, muscle fiber necrosis and regeneration, and occasionally mental retardation. Treatment includes prednisone (**Table 13**).

36.

B Rabies

Neg**r**i bodies occur in **r**abies, Lewy bodies in Parkinsonism, Hirano bodies in Alzheimer's, and Bunina bodies in ALS (**Table 10**).

37.

C Rarely cystic

Pilocytic astrocytomas contain Rosenthal fibers (*white arrow*), eosinophilic granular bodies (*black arrow*), and biphasic architecture with both cystic (C) and fascicular (F) patterns. Grossly, they are typically cystic with a mural nodule.

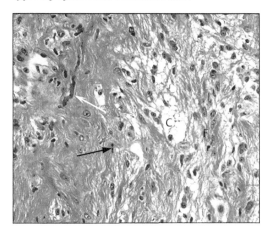

38.

E Canavan's disease

Macrocephaly is a feature of Canavan's, Alexander's, and Tay–Sachs diseases (**Table 12**).

39.

E Basilar tip

This left vertebral artery angiogram is showing a basilar tip aneurysm (*arrow*).

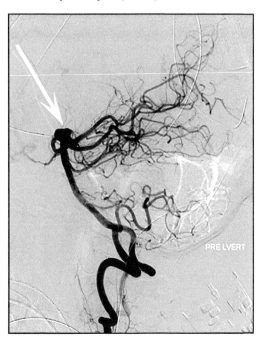

40.

C Amyotrophic lateral sclerosis (ALS)

Bunina bodies are seen in ALS (**Table 10**).

41.

C Glioblastoma multiforme (GBM)

These vascular endothelial proliferations are evidence of grade IV astrocytoma (GBM), usually associated with necrosis, nuclear atypia, and increased mitoses.

42.

B The other eye can't abduct

One-and-a-half syndrome is characterized by bilateral internuclear ophthalmoplegia resulting in bilateral failure of adduction, as well as VI nerve palsy on one side resulting in failure of abduction of that eye only. It is caused by bilateral lesion of medial longitudinal fasciculus, plus unilateral VI nerve palsy. Causes include brain stem ischemia or demyelination.

43.

D Corpus callosotomy

Typical indication for corpus callosotomy is drop attacks. It prevents spread of seizures to the contralateral hemisphere. Risks include disconnection syndrome; therefore, the posterior part of the corpus callosum (splenium) should be preserved.

44.

A PCOM (posterior communicating artery)

A PCOM aneurysm (*arrow*) is seen on this angiogram.

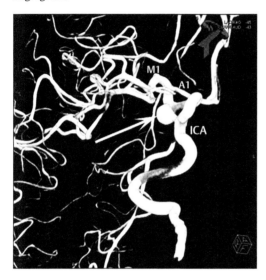

45.

B Multiple sclerosis (MS)

Typical clinical picture and imaging for MS. The T2 flair signals (hyperintense, triangular, and perpendicular to the lateral ventricle) are called Dawson's fingers. The patient needs a lumbar puncture to look for oligoclonal bands. Treatment includes corticosteroids, plasmapheresis, and disease-modifying agents including interferon and ocrelizumab.

46.

E 22

Schwannomas contain compact areas called Antoni A (A) and loose areas called Antoni **B** (**b**lasted apart; B). Verocay bodies (V) have nuclear palisading around anuclear areas. Some nuclei are arranged like a school of fish (S). They can occur in NF2, which is inherited as autosomal dominant on chromosome 22.

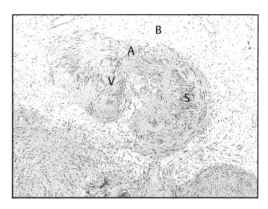

47.

C A synovial cyst

Synovial cysts are hyperintense on T2 MRI and are associated with the facet joints. In this case, it compresses the traversing left L5 nerve root causing radiculopathy. Occasionally, they present with neurogenic claudication. Dynamic X-rays are helpful to look for instability. If patients fail conservative measures, surgical treatment includes decompression with or without fusion, depending on the presence or absence of instability, respectively.

48.

A Meningioma

A calcified psammoma body is seen in the center. Whorls are also present, confirming the diagnosis of **men**ingioma. These tumors are positive for **EM**A and Vi**men**tin and may occur in patients with NF2.

49.

A Ependymoma

Cervical spinal cord expansion maximum at C5–C6 suggests an intramedullary tumor. Syringomyelia would have the same signal as CSF. Edema and hemosiderin deposition at both ends may show as a cap sign and are suggestive of ependymoma. The goal of surgery is gross total resection.

50.

C Low flow

Spinal AVMs types I and IV are high flow low pressure and present with venous hypertension, while types II and III are high flow high pressure and present with hemorrhage (**Table 17**). Surgery for type I includes laminectomy and intradural obliteration of the draining vein.

Further Reading: Borden JA, Wu JK, Shucart WA. A proposed classification for spinal and cranial dural arteriovenous fistulous malformations and implications for treatment. *J Neurosurg.* 1995 Feb;82(2):166–179

51.

B Guillain–Mollaret triangle

Guillain–Mollaret triangle is composed of dentate, red, and inferior olivary nuclei. Injury causes oculopalatal myoclonus (**Fig. 11**).

52.

E Anti-VGCC (voltage-gated calcium channel)

LEMS is caused by antibodies against presynaptic VCCC and occurs in small cell lung cancer. Anti-H*u* also occurs in small cell l*u*ng cancer and causes peripheral ne*u*ropathy. Anti-Tr occurs in Hodgkin's lymphoma and affects anterior horn cells and cerebellum. Anti-Ri occurs in breast cancer and causes opsoclonus. Myasthenia gravis is caused by antibodies against postsynaptic nicotinic AchR in the muscle (**Table 16, Fig. 26**).

53.

D Red nucleus

Benedikt's syndrome is a midbrain stroke syndrome involving the third cranial n causing ipsilateral IIIrd n palsy and red nucleus causing contralateral ataxia. Weber's syndrome involves ipsilateral IIIrd n palsy and contralateral hemiplegia (corticospinal tract) (**Fig. 13**).

54.

E Shunt for hydrocephalus

Fibrillary astrocytoma (grade II) features increased cellularity without mitoses, necrosis, or endothelial proliferation. The tumor is GFAP positive. Tectal gliomas are self-limited; they tend not to grow and do not require surgical resection. If they cause obstructive hydrocephalus, they can be treated by CSF diversion through shunting or endoscopic third ventriculostomy.

55.

D Keratin

Schwannomas are S100 positive. Diffuse keratin is found in epidermoid and dermoid cysts. Focal keratin is found in craniopharyngioma (sellar and suprasellar), adamantinomatous type (**Table 8**).

56.

C Type II dens fracture

Os odontoideum is more circular with cortical bone all around, treatment is posterior C1–C2 fusion. Type I dens fracture involves the tip of the dens (apical/alar ligament avulsion) and can be treated in a collar; type III involves the body of C2 and usually heals in a collar. Type II (the presented CT) is at the base of the dens, when non-displaced can have a trial of a cervical collar, when displaced surgery should be considered since the rate of nonunion is high. They can be treated by an anterior odontoid screw if the anatomy is favorable, or posterior C1-C2 screws.

57.

A Pseudorosette

*P*seudorosettes are around *b*lood vessels and occur in e*p*endymomas. Flexner–Wintersteiner rosette occurs around a central canal and are seen in ependymoma, pineoblastoma, and retinoblastoma. Homer–Wright rosette occurs in medulloblastoma or PNET and has no central canal or blood vessel. Very large rosettes are seen in pineocytoma (**Table 7**).

58.

E Arylsulfatase A deficiency

Canavan's disease is caused by deficiency in N-acetyl-aspartoacylase. It is autosomal recessive, affects Ashkenasi Jews, involves U fibers, causes spongy white matter, markedly enlarged mitochondria, and N-acetyl aspartic aciduria. It presents with macrocephaly, mental retardation, and blindness (**Table 12**).

59.

B Ryanodine receptor

Malignant hyperthermia is inherited as autosomal dominant on chromosome 19q, caused by ryanodine receptor mutation. There is increased serum CK. Features include fever, rigidity, and hypertension. Treatment includes dantrolene (**Table 13**).

60.

C Macrocephaly

Macrocephaly is not a feature of Gaucher's disease. It occurs in Tay–Sachs, Alexander's, and Canavan's diseases (**Table 12**).

9 Test 5—Neurobiology and Critical Care

Amgad Hanna, Yiping Li, and Joshua Medow

1.

The neurotransmitter from the putamen to globus pallidus (GP) is

A. Dopamine
B. Acetylcholine
C. 5-hydroxytryptamine (5-HT)
D. Glutamate
E. Gamma aminobutyric acid (GABA)

2.

Increased pulmonary dead space occurs in

A. Pneumonia
B. Pulmonary edema
C. Pulmonary embolism
D. High altitudes
E. Pneumothorax

3.

Which of the following values of cerebral blood flow lies within the ischemic penumbra?

A. 1–5 mL/100 g/min
B. 10–20 mL/100 g/min
C. 25–35 mL/100 g/min
D. 40–50 mL/100 g/min
E. 50–55 mL/100 g/min

4.

Botulinum toxin blocks

A. Adrenergic receptors
B. Nicotinic acetylcholine receptors
C. Muscarinic acetylcholine receptors
D. Acetylcholine release at the neuromuscular junction
E. Acetylcholine degradation

5.

Which receptors are found in the dermal papillae of the finger tips, are rapidly adapting, and are responsible for touch sensation?

A. Meissner's corpuscles
B. Pacinian corpuscles
C. Ruffini end organs
D. Free nerve endings
E. Hair end organs

6.

A 72-year-old man is admitted for osteomyelitis and discitis. He has a history of severe chronic obstructive pulmonary disease (COPD) and presents with fever, confusion, respiratory distress, leg pain, and weakness. He has a history of heavy smoking. An ABG shows: pH 7.23, PCO_2 72 mmHg, PO_2 91 mmHg, and HCO_3 28 mEq/L. What is the most likely diagnosis?

A. Compensated respiratory acidosis
B. Respiratory acidosis and metabolic acidosis
C. Respiratory acidosis with incomplete metabolic compensation
D. Metabolic acidosis with incomplete respiratory compensation
E. Metabolic acidosis

7.

A 15-year-old girl with sickle cell disease presents with acute right leg weakness. A head CT was performed which shows a small stroke in the ACA territory. The patient recovers well and visits you in clinic having fully recovered. Which of the following interventions reduces the frequency of sickle cell crisis?

A. Antibiotics
B. Hydroxyurea
C. Regular blood transfusions
D. Erythropoietin
E. Splenectomy

8.

The most excitable part of a neuron is

A. The dendrites
B. The cell body (soma)
C. The axon hillock
D. The axon at the nodes of Ranvier
E. The axon in-between the nodes of Ranvier

9.

Neuronal depolarization is caused by

A. Potassium influx
B. Calcium influx
C. Chloride efflux
D. Sodium efflux
E. Sodium influx

10.

The optic n fibers arise from which cells?

A. Bipolar
B. Amacrine
C. Horizontal
D. Ganglion
E. Rods and cones

11.

On an EEG, if the δ waves constitute >50%, this pattern is consistent with

A. Awake quiet
B. Stage 1 sleep
C. Stage 2 sleep
D. Stage 3 sleep
E. Stage 4 sleep

12.

All of the following drugs increase the effect of warfarin (Coumadin), *except*

A. Barbiturates
B. Benzodiazepines
C. Bactrim (trimethoprim)
D. Cimetidine
E. Salicylates

13.

A 17-year-old girl with sickle cell disease presents with a small acute right MCA stroke. What is the most important treatment to reduce morbidity and mortality?

A. Exchange transfusion
B. Aspirin
C. Hydroxyurea
D. Folic acid
E. Erythropoietin

14.

Which anesthetic decreases cerebral blood flow?

A. Isofluorane
B. Ketamine
C. Thiopental
D. Nitrous oxide
E. Halothane

15.

Red man syndrome can be a side effect of which antibiotic?

A. Penicillin
B. Vancomycin
C. Cephalosporins
D. Aminoglycosides
E. Imipenem

16.

A 23-year-old obese woman presents with progressive blindness over the past week. Recent ophthalmologic examination reveals grade 3 papilledema and an afferent pupillary defect (APD) in the right eye with 20/200 vision in the left eye. The patient undergoes a diagnostic angiogram. Which venous structure is identified by the *arrow*?

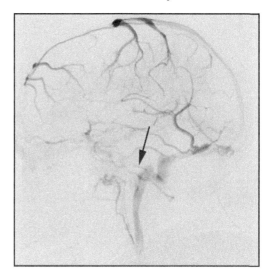

A. Superior sagittal sinus
B. Superior petrosal sinus
C. Inferior sagittal sinus
D. Inferior petrosal sinus
E. Thalamostriate vein

17.

The same patient was subsequently evaluated with a dedicated venogram which reveals the following findings (*arrow*). Which intervention can help predict success after transverse sinus stenting?

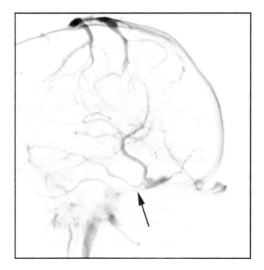

A. Weight loss
B. Acetazolamide (Diamox) therapy
C. Manometry across the site of stenosis
D. Heparin drip
E. Coumadin

18.

Gelastic seizures are typically observed with

A. Hypothalamic hamartomas
B. Tectal gliomas
C. Dysembryoplastic neuroepithelial tumors (DNET)
D. Subependymal giant cell astrocytoma (SEGA)
E. Ganglioglioma

19.

The main neurotransmitter output of the locus ceruleus is

A. Serotonin
B. Glutamate
C. GABA (gamma-amino butyric acid)
D. Norepinephrine (NE)
E. Acetylcholine

20.

Clarke's nucleus gives origin to the

A. Ventral spinothalamic tract
B. Lateral spinothalamic tract
C. Ventral spinocerebellar tract
D. Dorsal spinocerebellar tract
E. Spino-olivary tract

21.

Internuclear ophthalmoplegia (INO) is caused by a lesion of the

A. Medial forebrain bundle (MFB)
B. Medial longitudinal fasciculus (MLF)
C. Diagonal band of Broca (DBB)
D. Stria terminalis
E. Indusium griseum

22.

Klüver–Bucy syndrome is associated with bilateral damage of

A. Amygdala
B. Hippocampus
C. Fornix
D. Lateral hypothalamic nuclei
E. Thalamic fasciculus

23.

Vision occurs when metarhodopsin 2 activates

A. cAMP
B. G protein
C. Calcium channels
D. Acetylcholine receptors
E. Potassium channels

24.

Concerning the muscle spindle, the nuclear bag fibers have all of the following characteristics, *except*

A. Dynamic firing
B. Tonic firing
C. Central location
D. Annulospiral ending
E. Flower-spray ending

25.

All of the following is true about Na valproate, *except*

A. Decreases Na conductance
B. Can be hepatotoxic
C. Can be teratogenic (myelo-meningocele)
D. Can cause tremors
E. Can cause polycystic ovarian disease

26.

Spike-dome waves on EEG at 3 Hz are observed in

A. Lennox–Gastaut syndrome
B. Grand mal seizures
C. Absence seizures
D. REM sleep
E. Stage 4 sleep

27.

Which drug has no positive inotropic effect (β_1)?

A. Dopamine
B. Dobutamine
C. Epinephrine
D. Phenylephrine (Neosynephrine)
E. Norepinephrine (Levophed)

28.

A 42-year-old otherwise healthy man presents for an elective microdiscectomy for L5 radiculopathy. The patient undergoes general anesthesia and his ventilation is on a volume control mode. During surgery, ABG shows: pH 7.22, PCO_2 70 mmHg, PO_2 92 mmHg, and HCO_3 27 mEq/L. The best next step is

A. Increase the respiratory rate
B. Decrease the tidal volume
C. Change the mode of ventilation to pressure support
D. Increase the FiO_2
E. Cancel the surgery

29.

A 33-year-old otherwise healthy woman presents for an elective craniotomy. The patient undergoes general anesthesia and her ventilation is under pressure-regulated volume control (PRVC). During surgery, an ABG was sent and shows: pH 7.52, PCO_2 20 mmHg, PO_2 92 mmHg, and HCO_3 22 mEq/L. What is the diagnosis?

A. Respiratory alkalosis
B. Respiratory acidosis
C. Metabolic alkalosis
D. Metabolic acidosis
E. Mixed respiratory and metabolic acidosis

30.

A 72-year-old man presents with chest pain, syncope, dizziness, vertigo, and headache. He is admitted to the hospital where telemetry reveals intermittent episodes of bradycardia and tachycardia. What is the most likely diagnosis?

A. Supraventricular tachycardia
B. Atrial flutter
C. Atrial fibrillation
D. Sick sinus syndrome
E. Vasovagal episode

31.

A 22-year-old man with bacterial endocarditis due to IV drug use presents with headache, confusion, and left arm weakness. He is admitted to the hospital where a head CT reveals a right parietal mass with surrounding edema. An abscess is suspected. What is the most likely bacterial agent?

A. *Viridans streptococci*
B. *Enterococci*
C. *Staphylococcus aureus*
D. *Escherichia coli*
E. *Pseudomonas*

32.

A 60-year-old woman with uncontrolled hypertension presents with acute onset right-sided weakness, aphasia, and left gaze preference. He was last seen well the evening prior to presentation. On examination, the patient has GCS of 7 and the left pupil is dilated and poorly reactive. The head CT shows a large left-sided MCA infarct. Which of the following measures most effectively reduces mortality?

A. IV mannitol 1 g/kg
B. Hyperventilation
C. IV tPA
D. Hemicraniectomy
E. Mechanical thrombectomy

33.

A 62-year-old diabetic woman presents with acute onset left-sided weakness, with last known well 6 hours prior to presentation. The head CT shows a hyperdense right MCA sign with areas of hypodensity in the basal ganglia and insula. The CT perfusion imaging reveals a large area of prolonged mean transit time, reduced cerebral blood flow, but maintained cerebral blood volume. Which of the following measures has been shown to reduce mortality?

A. IV Mannitol 1 g/kg
B. Hyperventilation
C. IV tPA
D. Hemicraniectomy
E. Mechanical thrombectomy

34.

A 13-year-old boy with sickle cell disease presents with acute left arm weakness. A head CT was performed which shows a small stroke in the MCA territory involving the internal capsule and basal ganglia. His blood pressure is 130/79, blood glucose is 152 mg/dL, and sodium of 140 mEq/L. CTA was normal. The patient recovers well and visits you in clinic after having fully recovered. Which of the following interventions will reduce his risk for further strokes?

A.   Encephaloduroarteriosynagiosis (EDAS)
B.   Aspirin
C.   Adequate hydration
D.   Insulin
E.   Antihypertensive medications

35.

A 29-year-old female is postpartum day 1 from a normal uncomplicated delivery. She received epidural anesthesia during delivery and developed a post procedure CSF leak with headaches especially in an upright position. By day 2 she was scheduled to discharge but she was more obtunded in the afternoon and was difficult to arouse. A head CT was performed which reveals an intraparenchymal hemorrhage, cerebral edema, and multiple dilated vessels at the vertex. What is the most likely diagnosis?

A.   Dural arterial venous fistula
B.   Arteriovenous malformation
C.   Cerebral sinus thrombosis
D.   Brain sag syndrome
E.   Hemorrhagic Encephalitis

36.

For the above patient, what is the treatment of choice?

A.   Craniotomy for decompression
B.   Heparin drip
C.   Endovascular treatment
D.   Stereotactic Radiation
E.   IV hydration

37.

A 65-year-old man involved in an MVC was diagnosed with an aortic injury. He became hemodynamically unstable and was taken to surgery for an exploratory laparotomy. Postoperatively he is weak in the lower extremities. The most appropriate next step is

A.   MRI of the lumbar spine
B.   MRI of the head
C.   Reduce mean arterial blood pressure
D.   Blood transfusion
E.   Placement of a lumbar drain

38.

A 34-year-old woman presents with hypotension and a sodium of 124 mEq/L. On examination, she is a thin and tan woman who appears lethargic and is hypotensive. She notes having recent weight loss and loss of appetite but is otherwise neurologically intact. Which of the following should be suspected?

A.   Addison's disease
B.   Alcoholism
C.   Congestive heart failure
D.   SIADH
E.   Hypothyroidism

39.

A 3-year-old boy was abused and presents with multiple skull base fractures after non-accidental trauma and has a CSF leak. He develops meningitis 5 days later and antibiotics are initiated. What is the most likely causative agent?

A.   *Staphylococcus aureus*
B.   *Escherichia coli*
C.   *Streptococcus pneumoniae*
D.   *Listeria monocytogenes*
E.   *Enterococcus*

40.

A 3-year-old boy is being treated for a pseudomonas infection with antibiotics. A week after initiation of treatment he begins to develop renal failure secondary to non-oliguric acute tubular necrosis. Which of the following antibiotics is the likely cause?

A.   Cefuroxime
B.   Penicillin
C.   Tetracycline
D.   Tobramycin
E.   Bactrim

41.

A 14-year-old boy with sickle cell disease presents with acute left arm weakness. A head CT was performed which shows a small stroke in the right MCA territory. CTA was within normal limits. Which of the following follow-up studies should be performed annually?

A. Transcranial Doppler
B. CTA
C. Digital subtraction angiography
D. MRI of the head
E. MRA of the head

42.

Which of the following is *not* a Vitamin K–dependent clotting factor?

A. Factor II
B. Factor V
C. Factor VII
D. Factor IX
E. Factor X

43.

Which of the following neurotransmitter receptors is associated with Ca^{++} influx and cell death?

A. Nor-epinephrine
B. Glutamate
C. Serotonin
D. Dopamine
E. GABA

44.

Which of the following nerve fiber types transmits prickling pain and temperature?

A. Ia
B. Ib
C. II
D. III
E. IV

45.

Which of the following thalamic nuclei is associated with the spinothalamic tracts?

A. Ventral anterior
B. Medial dorsal
C. VPLc (ventral posterolateral, pars caudalis)
D. Pulvinar
E. Medial geniculate

46.

Which Brodmann's area of the somatosensory cortex is associated with deep pressure and joint position?

A. 1
B. 2
C. 3a
D. 3b
E. 4

47.

A 65-year-old man was diagnosed with an aortic dissection and was taken emergently to surgery for vascular repair. Surgery went uncomplicated but postoperatively the patient becomes paraplegic. What treatment strategies could have prevented these symptoms?

A. MRI of the lumbar spine prior to surgery
B. MRI of the head prior to surgery
C. Reduce mean arterial blood pressure
D. Blood transfusion
E. Distal bypass during surgery

48.

Which Rexed lamina represents the second-order neuron for fast pain transmission?

A. Lamina I
B. Lamina II
C. Lamina III
D. Lamina IV
E. Lamina V

49.

Which of the following is *not* a side effect of DBS of the periaqueductal gray for treatment of chronic pain?

A. Diplopia
B. Oscillopsia
C. Fear
D. Dysphagia
E. Anxiety

50.

Which of the following is *false* regarding G protein receptors in phototransduction?

A. Metarhodopsin 2 activates G protein receptors
B. The alpha subunit binds GTP
C. cGMP converts to 5′ GMP
D. There is increased current through Na channels
E. It results in an electric-graded conduction

51.
Which of the following nerve fiber type is associated with muscle spindles, annulospiral type?

A. Ia
B. Ib
C. II
D. III
E. IV

52.
Which of the following cells provide lateral inhibition to increase contrast in phototransduction?

A. Retinal cells
B. Horizontal cells
C. Bipolar cells
D. Amacrine cells
E. Ganglion cells

53.
Which optic pathway projection transmits to the basal brain for behavioral functions?

A. Suprachiasmatic nucleus
B. Pretectal nucleus
C. Superior colliculus
D. Ventral lateral geniculate body (LGB)
E. Dorsal lateral geniculate body

54.
A 16-year-old boy attends a loud concert. When he comes home his mother notices that he yells whenever he speaks and she suspects he is having hearing difficulty. The muscle involved in a reflex that protects the cochlea by attenuating loud sounds is

A. Muller's
B. Short ciliary
C. Tensor veli palatini
D. Stapedius
E. Posterior belly of the digastric

55.
A 40-year-old man presents after a motorcycle accident. He is awake but unable to move his arms and legs and has no appreciable tone or reflexes. You suspect spinal shock. Which reflex is the first to return after conclusion of spinal shock?

A. Babinski
B. Hoffman
C. Suprapatellar
D. Abdominal
E. Bulbocavernosus (Osinski)

56.
A 37-year-old female presents to the ER after being found down outside a bar in the early morning. A head CT revealed a large intraparenchymal hemorrhage. She is extensor posturing. Which of the following nuclei is associated with this reflex?

A. Cochlear nucleus
B. Superior vestibular
C. Inferior vestibular
D. Lateral vestibular
E. Medial vestibular

57.
Which of the following afferent tracts transmit motor, premotor, and sensory information from the pons to the contralateral cerebellar hemisphere?

A. Juxtarestiform body
B. Restiform body
C. Middle cerebellar peduncle
D. Superior cerebellar peduncle
E. Dorsal columns

58.
A newborn girl presents with tachypnea, hepatosplenomegaly, and ventriculomegaly. Diagnostic angiogram is shown below. Given the imaging findings (*arrow*), which of the following is the strongest determining factor for urgent endovascular intervention?

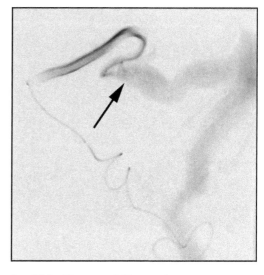

A. Risk of intracranial hemorrhage
B. Risk of seizures
C. Development of hydrocephalus
D. Renal failure
E. Heart failure

59.
A 37-year-old man presents after being ejected from a vehicle at high speed. He has a dilated pupil and was given 100 g mannitol IV immediately prior to arriving at your hospital. He has a serum sodium of 131 mEq/L. The emergency medicine physician who is evaluating him is concerned about pseudo-hyponatremia. All of the following would lead to pseudohyponatremia, *except*

A. Elevated BUN (blood urea nitrogen)
B. Elevated serum glucose
C. Mannitol
D. 0.45% saline
E. Hyperproteinemia

60.
A 45-year-old man presents with a history of elevated ICP treated with 3% hypertonic saline. The critical care nurse obtains an ABG which shows: pH 7.31, PCO_2 40 mmHg, PO_2 92 mmHg, and HCO_3 17 mEq/L. The basic metabolic panel shows serum Na 140 mEq/L, Cl 116 mEq/L, and HCO_3 17 mEq/L. What is the most likely diagnosis?

A. Methanol Poisoning
B. Ethylene Glycol Poisoning
C. Hyperchloremia
D. Uremia
E. Salicylate Poisoning

10 Answer Key 5

Amgad Hanna, Yiping Li, and Joshua Medow

1.

E Gamma aminobutyric acid (GABA)

GABA and enkephalins are neurotransmitters from putamen to GPe, GABA and substance P from putamen to GPi. Dopamine is from substantia nigra pars compacta to striatum (defective in Parkinson's disease) while Ach from amygdala to cortex (defective in Alzheimer's disease), from cortex to caudate, and from caudate to putamen. Serotonin (5-HT) is from dorsal raphe nucleus to substantia nigra and striatum (involved in non-REM sleep) while glutamate is from thalamus to striatum and cortex, from cortex to putamen and subthalamic nucleus, and from subthalamic nucleus to GPe, GPi, and substantia nigra (**Fig. 7**).

2.

C Pulmonary embolism

Pulmonary embolism causes a ventilation-perfusion mismatch where the vessels are occluded causing a dead space effect. When the alveoli are filled with fluid as in pulmonary edema or pneumonia, a shunt effect occurs.

3.

B 10–20 mL/100 g/min

While the normal cerebral blood flow is 50 mL/100 g/min, with higher flow in the gray matter, the ischemic penumbra occurs at 8–23 mL/100 g/min.

4.

D Acetylcholine release at the neuromuscular junction

Botulinum toxin degrades SNARE proteins at the neuromuscular junction. The SNARE (SNAP receptor) complex are essential for acetylcholine release and are composed of: synaptobrevin, syntaxin, and SNAP-25 (synaptosomal-associated protein-25 kDa) (**Fig. 26**).

5.

A Meissner's corpuscles

Meissner's corpuscles are found in the dermal papillae of the finger tips and lips, transmit touch and vibration through type II fibers, are rapidly adapting, and have a small receptive field (**Table 2**).

6.

C Respiratory acidosis with incomplete metabolic compensation

In chronic respiratory acidosis due to COPD, the kidneys respond by retaining HCO_3 (renal compensation). The expected HCO_3 should be: 4 mEq/L for every 10 mmHg increase in PCO_2. This patient has a mild metabolic alkalosis that is not completely compensating for the respiratory acidosis noted on the blood gas, indicating that the PCO_2 is not chronically elevated enough to drive a significant increase in HCO_3.

7.

B Hydroxyurea

Hydroxyurea increases fetal hemoglobin and decreases platelets and leukocytes, thereby reducing the frequency of sickling and need for blood transfusions after acute crisis.

8.

C The axon hillock

The axon hillock is the most excitable part of a neuron. It has a high concentration of Na^+ channels, a resting membrane potential of –65 mV, and a threshold for action potential of –45 mV. This is usually where the action potential starts.

Further Reading: Kole MH, Stuart GJ. Signal processing in the axon initial segment. *Neuron* 2012;73(2):235–247

9.

E Sodium influx

During the neuronal action potential, the depolarization is caused by opening of Na^+ channels and Na^+ influx, while repolarization is caused by closure of Na^+ channels (inner inactivation gate) and K^+ efflux. At rest, the inactivation gate is open and the outer activation gate is closed. Tetrodotoxin and saxitoxin block Na^+ channels and so do local anesthetics and some seizure medications (phenytoin and carbamazepine) (**Fig. 27**).

Further Reading: Platkiewicz J, Brette R. A threshold equation for action potential initiation. *PLoS Comput Biol.* 2010;6(7):e1000850

10.

D Ganglion

In the retina, the signal is transmitted from the rods and cones to the bipolar cells to the ganglion cells, whose axons make the optic n (**Fig. 30**).

11.

E Stage 4 sleep

During sleep: Stage 1 is characterized by low-voltage α waves, stage 2 K complexes and sleep spindles, stage 3 some δ waves as well as K complexes and sleep spindles, stage 4 δ waves >50%, and REM sleep β waves. Awake quiet features α waves and awake alert β waves (**Fig. 31**).

12.

A Barbiturates

Barbiturates, phenytoin, and carbamazepine stimulate liver microsomal enzymes, and therefore increase the degradation of Coumadin. Benzodiazepines, Bactrim, and cimetidine are liver inhibitors, therefore increase the effect of Coumadin, with increased risk of bleeding. Salicylates displace Coumadin from its protein-binding sites in the blood, thus increasing its effect (**Fig. 32**).

13.

A Exchange transfusion

Blood transfusions decrease the morbidity and mortality in patients with sickle cell crisis, especially with pulmonary and central nervous system complications. Exchange transfusion is even more effective in reducing the level of HgbS by taking out the patient's own blood and transfusing a donor's blood. This reduces the risk of vaso-occlusive disease.

Further Reading: Adams RJ, McKie VC, Hsu L, et al. Prevention of a first stroke by transfusions in children with sickle cell anemia and abnormal results on transcranial Doppler ultrasonography. *N Engl J Med.* 1998;339(1):5–11

14.

C Thiopental

Thiopental, etomidate, and fentanyl decrease cerebral blood flow. Nitrous oxide, isoflurane, ketamine, enflurane, and halothane increase cerebral blood flow (***Nike Halo***).

15.

B Vancomycin

Red man syndrome can be associated with rapid infusion of vancomycin. It is characterized by erythematous rash and pruritus in the upper body, head, and neck with possible hypotension. Treat with anti-histamines.

16.

D Inferior petrosal sinus

The patient has a clinical picture of pseudotumor cerebri. The inferior petrosal sinus courses along the petroclival fissure and connects the cavernous sinus anteromedially to the jugular bulb posterolaterally (**Fig. 5**).

17.

C Manometry across the site of stenosis

The *arrow* points to transverse sinus stenosis. Manometry across the site of stenosis with significant pressure differentials is a positive predictor of success after transverse sinus stenting. Weight loss and Diamox are viable treatment options for pseudotumor cerebri.

Further Readings: Ahmed RM, Wilkinson M, Parker GD, et al. Transverse sinus stenting for idiopathic intracranial hypertension: a review of 52 patients and of model predictions. *AJNR AM J Neuroradiol.* 2011;32(8):1408–1414

Bussière M, Falero R, Nicolle D, Proulx A, Patel V, Pelz D. Unilateral transverse sinus stenting of patients with idiopathic intracranial hypertension. *AJNR Am J Neuroradiol.* 2010;31(4):645–650

Kumpe DA, Bennett JL, Seinfeld J, Pelak VS, Chawla A, Tierney M. Dural sinus stent placement for idiopathic intracranial hypertension. *J Neurosurg.* 2012;116(3):538–548

18.

A Hypothalamic hamartomas

Gelastic seizures manifest as a sudden burst of laughter. Hypothalamic hamartomas are characterized by gelastic seizures, precocious puberty, and developmental delay.

19.

D Nor-epinephrine (NE)

The main output of locus ceruleus is NE and it is responsible for REM sleep (**Figs. 7 and 31**).

20.

D Dorsal spinocerebellar tract

Clarke's nucleus is present in lamina VII of the spinal cord gray matter (C8–L2) and conveys proprioception from the lower extremities. It forms the uncrossed dorsal spinocerebellar tract that travels through the inferior cerebellar peduncle (**Figs. 11 and 15**).

21.

B Medial longitudinal fasciculus (MLF)

INO is caused by a lesion of the MLF and causes inability of the ipsilateral eye to adduct, while the normal side abducts. **P**osterior INO is caused by a **p**ontine lesion and has **p**reserved convergence. Anterior INO is caused by a midbrain lesion and has decreased convergence.

22.

A Amygdala

Klüver–Bucy syndrome is associated with bilateral damage of the amygdala. It causes hyperorality, hyperphagia, hypersexuality, amnesia, tameness, and visual agnosia.

23.

B G protein

Light converts retinal rhodopsin into metarhodopsin 2. The latter activates G protein, which stimulates phosphodiesterase, thus converting cGMP to 5'GMP. Na^+ channels close, resulting in hyperpolarization and a graded electric conduction (**Fig. 30**).

24.

E Flower-spray ending

The intrafusal muscle fibers of the muscle spindle are responsible for proprioception. The nuclear bag fibers are larger, dynamic, tonic, central, with primary annulospiral endings, carried by type Ia fibers (120 m/s). The nuclear **c**hain fibers are **s**maller, **s**tatic, tonic, e**cc**entric, with primary annulo**s**piral and **s**econdary flower-**s**pray endings, carried by type II fibers, traveling at thirty to **s**eventy m/s (**Table 3**).

25.

A Decreases Na conductance

Concerning the mechanism of action of antiepileptic drugs: Na valproate increases GABA, benzodiazepines and barbiturates stimulate $GABA_A$ receptors, while phenytoin and carbamazepine decrease Na conductance by blocking Na channels (**Table 34, Figs. 26 and 27**).

Further Reading: Henschel O, Gipson KE, Bordey A. $GABA_A$ receptors, anesthetics and anticonvulsants in brain development. *CNS Neurol Disord Drug Targets* 2008 Apr;7(2):211–224

26.

C Absence seizures

Spike-dome waves at 1–2 Hz are characteristic of Lennox–Gastaut syndrome, at 3 Hz absence seizures, at 4–6 Hz juvenile myoclonic epilepsy (**Fig. 31**).

27.

D Phenylephrine (Neosynephrine)

Phenylephrine is predominantly α stimulant, isoproterenol β, NE $α_1$ $α_2$ $β_1$, and epinephrine $α_1$ $α_2$ $β_1$ $β_2$ (**Table 33, Fig. 25**).

28.

A Increase the respiratory rate

The patient is suffering from acute respiratory acidosis due to hypoventilation. HCO_3 increase is as expected, 1 mEq/L for every 10 mmHg increase in PCO_2; therefore, there is no associated metabolic component. This is due to reduced expiration of PCO_2, and therefore increasing the respiratory rate or tidal volume would correct this problem.

29.

A Respiratory alkalosis

The patient has a pure respiratory alkalosis from hyperventilation.

30.

D Sick sinus syndrome

Sick sinus syndrome is due to dysfunction of the SA (sinoatrial) node and is commonly seen in the elderly. It often manifests as periods of intermittent bradycardia and tachycardia on cardiac rhythms.

31.

C *Staphylococcus aureus*

Staphylococcus aureus is the most common causative organism in the majority of bacterial endocarditis cases especially those associated with IV drug abuse.

32.

D Hemicraniectomy

Surgical decompression has been shown to reduce the mortality of patients with malignant cerebral edema after a large territory infarct. Hyperventilation and mannitol are temporizing. Thrombectomy should not be performed as the infarction has been completed.

Further Reading: Vahedi K, Hofmeijer J, Juettler E, et al. Early decompressive surgery in malignant infarction of the middle cerebral artery: a pooled analysis of three randomised controlled trials. *Lancet Neurol.* 2007; 6(3): 215–222

33.

E   Mechanical thrombectomy

Thrombectomy has been shown to be effective in reducing mortality and improving functional outcomes after acute large vessel occlusions. In cases of large territory penumbra, thrombectomy should be performed.

Further Reading: Berkhemer OA, Fransen PS, Beumer D, et al. A randomized trial of intraarterial treatment for acute ischemic stroke. *N Engl J Med.* 2015;372(1):11–20

Campbell BC, Mitchell PJ, Kleinig TJ, et al. Endovascular therapy for ischemic stroke with perfusion-imaging selection. *N Engl J Med.* 2015; 372(11):1009–1018

Goyal M, Demchuk AM, Menon BK, et al. Randomized assessment of rapid endovascular treatment of ischemic stroke. *N Engl J Med.* 2015;372(11):1019–1030

34.

C   Adequate hydration

Dehydration precipitates sickling of red blood cells and development of subsequent stroke.

35.

C   Cerebral sinus thrombosis

Postpartum females are at high risk for developing cerebral venous sinus thrombosis which should be suspected with severe headaches, cerebral hemorrhage (usually flame-shaped), and cerebral edema.

36.

B   Heparin drip

Despite intracranial hemorrhage, anticoagulation with heparin is the treatment of choice because it reduces the venous outflow obstruction, thereby reducing cerebral edema. Endovascular therapy is used only as a last resort.

37.

E   Placement of a lumbar drain

Placement of a lumbar drain reduces intrathecal hydrostatic pressure and therefore increases spinal cord perfusion. Increasing the MAP can also be helpful.

38.

A   Addison's disease

Addison's disease presents with hypotension, hyponatremia, hyperkalemia, and skin hyperpigmentation (the precursor of ACTH also produces MSH which increases melanin on the skin).

39.

C   *Streptococcus pneumoniae*

Streptococcus pneumoniae is the most common pathogen after skull base fractures and meningitis. A third-generation cephalosporin is usually effective for treatment.

40.

D   Tobramycin

Tobramycin is an aminoglycoside and frequently causes acute tubular necrosis in addition to hearing loss and vestibular dysfunction. Vancomycin is also nephrotoxic and ototoxic.

41.

A   Transcranial Doppler

Patients are recommended to be evaluated with transcranial Dopplers annually for preventive management of stroke. Exchange transfusions should be considered when there is an abnormal finding on ultrasound.

Further Reading: Adams RJ, McKie VC, Hsu L, et al. Prevention of a first stroke by transfusions in children with sickle cell anemia and abnormal results on transcranial Doppler ultrasonography. *N Engl J Med.* 1998;339(1):5–11

42.

B   Factor V

Vitamin K–dependent clotting factors are II (prothrombin), VII, IX, X, protein C and S.

43.

B   Glutamate

The NMDA receptor which is inhibited by magnesium and activated by glutamate is associated with calcium influx and regulates cell death. It is both voltage-gated and ligand-gated. The non-NMDA receptors (kainate) are only ligand-gated and can also be implicated in cell death (**Fig. 26**).

Further Reading: Sattler R, Tymianski M. Molecular mechanisms of glutamate receptor-mediated excitotoxic neuronal cell death. *Mol Neurobiol.* 2001 Aug-Dec;24(1-3):107–129

44.

D III

Type III fibers (Aδ) are associated with sharp pain and temperature (cold) transmission. Type IV fibers (C) are associated with burning pain and temperature (cold and heat) sensation (**Table 1**).

45.

C VPLc (ventral posterolateral, pars caudalis)

The spinothalamic tracts relay in the VPLc, the latter projects to the sensory cortex (areas 3,1,2). The ventral spinothalamic tract also relays in the intralaminar nuclei and the periaqueductal gray (**Fig. 8**).

46.

B 2

Brodmann's area 4 is the motor cortex, 3a is for muscle and tendon stretch, 3b is for skin receptors (slow and rapid adapting), 1 is for rapid adapting skin (fine touch), and 2 pressure and joint position (**Fig. 1**).

47.

E Distal bypass during surgery

Distal bypass during aortic repair can restore spinal cord perfusion during cross clamping of the aorta. Lumbar drain or increasing MAPs can also be helpful.

48.

A Lamina I

Lamina I (marginal zone) transmits fast (sharp) pain while lamina II (substantia gelatinosa) transmits slow (burning) pain (**Fig. 15**).

49.

D Dysphagia

Dysphagia can result in dysfunction of the lower cranial nerves. The periaqueductal gray is at the level of the midbrain and is unlikely to result in dysphagia.

50.

D There is increased current through Na channels

Decreased current through the cGMP activated Na$^+$ channels, resulting in hyperpolarization. Light converts retinal rhodopsin into metarhodopsin 2. The latter activates G protein, which stimulates phosphodiesterase, thus converting cGMP to 5'GMP. Na$^+$ channels close, resulting in hyperpolarization and a graded electric conduction (**Fig. 30**).

51.

A Ia

Both type Ia (Aα) and II (Aβ,γ) fibers are associated with transmission of neuronal signals arising from the muscle spindle, the former for annulospiral and the latter for flower-spray. Type Ib is associated with Golgi tendon organ, III sharp pain and γ motor neuron, and type IV burning pain (**Table 1, Fig. 28**).

52.

B Horizontal cells

Horizontal cells transmit signals horizontally and laterally inhibit other cells to increase contrast.

53.

D Ventral lateral geniculate body (LGB)

Ventral LGB (magnocellular, layers 1 and 2) projects to the basal brain for behavioral functions. Both ventral and dorsal (parvocellular, layers 3–6) LGB project to the primary visual cortex (area 17). Superior colliculus is involved in conjugate eye movements, pretectal nucleus is associated with pupillary reflexes, and the suprachiasmatic nucleus regulates the circadian rhythm.

54.

D Stapedius

The stapedius muscle (supplied by VII) and tensor tympani (supplied by V) are involved with the attenuation of loud noise to protect the auditory system (**Fig. 14**).

55.

E Bulbocavernosus (Osinski)

Osinski (bulbocavernosus) reflex involves anal sphincter contraction in response to squeezing the glans or tugging on an indwelling urinary catheter. It is the first to return after spinal shock.

56.

D Lateral vestibular

Lateral vestibular nucleus (Dieter's) is involved with extensor posturing and is inhibited by the Purkinje cells of the anterior lobe of the cerebellum. This decerebrate rigidity also occurs due to loss of input from the rubrospinal tract.

57.

C Middle cerebellar peduncle

The superior and inferior (restiform body) cerebellar peduncles transmit information to the cerebellum from the spinal cord input rather than the cortex. Information from different areas of the cerebral cortex terminate in the ipsilateral pontine nuclei, then cross the midline to the contralateral cerebellar hemisphere through the middle cerebellar peduncle (**Fig. 11**).

58.

E Heart failure

Cardiac failure in choroidal type Vein of Galen malformations (*arrow*) is the strongest factor for determining timing of surgical intervention.

59.

D 0.45% saline

All answers except for D can cause a pseudohyponatremia, where the sodium level when corrected for the extra water brought into the vascular space by the osmotic load is otherwise normal. 0.45% saline can cause hyponatremia by directly diluting the sodium level and thus is not a pseudohyponatremia.

60.

C Hyperchloremia

The anion gap $= Na^+ - (Cl^- + HCO_3^-) = 140 - (116 + 17) = 140 - 133 = 7$ mEq/L, which is normal (<12). The patient has metabolic acidosis (low pH, low HCO_3), non-anion gap. The other answers indicate an anion gap acidosis but hyperchloremia is the only non-gap acidosis. Causes of high **anion gap** acidosis: **MUD PILES**: methanol, uremia, diabetic ketoacidosis, paracetamol, isoniazid, lactic acidosis, ethylene glycol, and salicylates. Causes of *non-gap* acidosis: *USED CARP*: ureterostomy, small bowel fistula, excess Cl, diarrhea, carbonic anhydrase inhibitors, Addison's disease, renal tubular acidosis, and pancreatic fistula.

1.
Which of the following vasopressors has no beta stimulant effect?

A. Dopamine
B. Dobutamine
C. Epinephrine
D. Norepinephrine (Levophed)
E. Phenylephrine (Neosynephrine)

2.
An injury in the location marked by the *arrow* will most likely cause

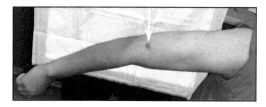

A. Claw hand
B. Benediction hand
C. Wrist drop
D. Froment's sign
E. Inability to make the OK sign

3.
Which anesthetic agent decreases cerebral blood flow?

A. Thiopental
B. Isofluorane
C. Ketamine
D. Nitrous oxide
E. Halothane

4.
The normal total blood volume of a normal full-term neonate is

A. 70 mL/kg
B. 75 mL/kg
C. 80 mL/kg
D. 90 mL/kg
E. 100 mL/kg

5.
Loop diuretics (Lasix) increase the serum value of

A. Potassium
B. Uric acid
C. Magnesium
D. Calcium
E. Chloride

6.
The total volume of cerebrospinal fluid (CSF) in a normal human is

A. 75 mL
B. 150 mL
C. 300 mL
D. 450 mL
E. None of the above

7.
If the patient experiences diplopia while placing DBS lead in the subthalamic nucleus (STN), the lead is too

A. Medial
B. Lateral
C. Anterior
D. Posterior
E. Deep

8.
Normal cerebral blood flow is

A. 25 mL/100 g/min
B. 50 mL/100 g/min
C. 75 mL/100 g/min
D. 100 mL/100 g/min

9.
Based on the following diagram, which number represents the internal cerebral v?

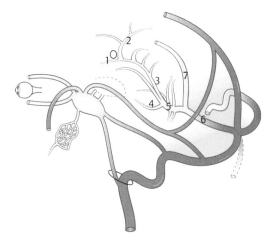

A. 1
B. 3
C. 4
D. 5
E. 6

10.

If the patient experiences phosphenes (flashing lights) while placing DBS lead in the globus pallidus internus (GPi), the lead is too

A. Medial
B. Lateral
C. Superficial
D. Deep
E. Anterior

11.

High anion gap acidosis is caused by all of the following, *except*

A. Accumulation of lactic acid
B. Diabetic ketoacidosis
C. Starvation
D. Increased serum beta-hydroxybutyrate
E. Diarrhea

12.

In the following figure, the fimbria of the fornix is represented by number

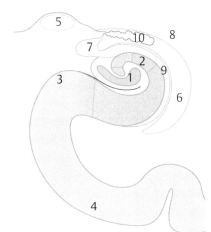

A. 1
B. 2
C. 3
D. 5
E. 7

13.

Which medication increases the risk of bleeding on Coumadin?

A. Benzodiazepines
B. Barbiturates
C. Carbamazepine
D. Rifampicin
E. Cholestyramine

14.

The ulnar n supplies all of the following muscles, *except*

A. Flexor carpi ulnaris
B. Abductor digiti minimi
C. Abductor pollicis brevis
D. Adductor pollicis
E. Interossei

15.

If the patient experiences contralateral gaze deviation while placing DBS lead in the subthalamic nucleus (STN), the lead should be moved

A. Medially
B. Laterally
C. Anteriorly
D. Deeper

16.

The positive predictive value of test A to detect disease X is

	Disease X present	Disease X absent
Test A +	80	20
Test A −	35	65

A. 65%
B. 69.6%
C. 76.5%
D. 80%

17.

Disseminated intravascular coagulation (DIC) is characterized by an increase in all of the following, *except*

A. Prothrombin time (PT)
B. Partial thromboplastin time (PTT)
C. Platelets
D. Fibrin degradation products (FDP)
E. Microvascular clots

18.

The main neurotransmitter of the thalamic fasciculus (Forel's Field H1 = FFH1) is

A. Gamma-aminobutyric acid (GABA)
B. Dopamine
C. 5-hydroxytryptamine (5-HT)
D. Glutamate
E. Acetylcholine

19.
The efferents of which thalamic nuclei connect to the cingulate cortex?

A.   Anterior nuclear group (ANG)
B.   Ventral anterior (VA)
C.   Lateral posterior (LP)
D.   Ventrolateral, pars oralis (VLo)
E.   Ventrolateral, pars caudalis (VLc)

20.
The use of which medication has been associated with cyanide toxicity?

A.   Nitroglycerin
B.   Sodium nitroprusside (Nipride)
C.   Nicardipine (Cardene)
D.   Nimodipine
E.   Labetalol

21.
Based on the following brachial plexus diagram, the ulnar n is represented by which number?

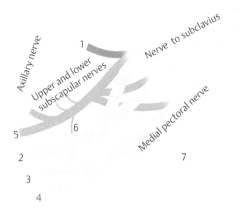

A.   1
B.   2
C.   3
D.   4
E.   5

22.
The Edinger–Westphal nucleus of the oculomotor n carries

A.   Special somatic afferents
B.   Special visceral afferents
C.   General somatic afferents
D.   General somatic efferents
E.   General visceral efferents

23.
The uncinate fasciculus carries crossed efferent fibers from which cerebellar nuclei?

A.   Fastigial
B.   Globose
C.   Emboliform
D.   Dentate

24.
Guillain–Mollaret triangle injury causes palatal myoclonus. Which nucleus is *not* part of the Guillain–Mollaret triangle?

A.   Red nucleus
B.   Inferior olivary nucleus
C.   Dentate nucleus
D.   Nucleus interpositus

25.
All of the following clotting factors are vitamin K–dependent, *except*

A.   II
B.   VII
C.   VIII
D.   IX
E.   X

26.
All of the following statements are true about Clarke's nucleus, *except* that

A.   It is located in the gray matter of the spinal cord.
B.   It spans spinal cord segments C8–L2.
C.   It conveys touch and proprioception.
D.   It sends efferents in the contralateral dorsal spinocerebellar tract.
E.   Efferents travel through the inferior cerebellar peduncle.

27.
The main neurotransmitter out of the locus ceruleus is

A.   Norepinephrine
B.   Acetylcholine
C.   Glutamate
D.   Dopamine
E.   Serotonin

28.

Which medication is the *least* beneficial in patients with asthma?

A. Beta blockers
B. Theophylline
C. Ipratropium
D. Steroids
E. Salbutamol

29.

Increased positive end-expiratory pressure (PEEP) results in all of the following, *except*

A. Barotrauma
B. Decreased cardiac output
C. Decreased shunt effect
D. Decreased dead space

30.

Which structure does *not* pass through the annulus of Zinn?

A. Cranial n III, superior division
B. Cranial n III, inferior division
C. Cranial n IV
D. Cranial n V, nasociliary branch
E. Cranial n VI

31.

Isoflurane causes anesthesia through

A. N-methyl-D-aspartate (NMDA)-receptor antagonism
B. Binding γ-aminobutyric acid type A (GABA$_A$) receptor
C. Na$^+$ channel blockade
D. Opioid agonism

32.

If the patient experiences dysarthria and muscle contractions while placing DBS lead in the nucleus ventralis intermedius (Vim), the lead is too

A. Medial
B. Lateral
C. Anterior
D. Posterior
E. Deep

33.

The medial forebrain bundle connects the septal nuclei to

A. Hypothalamus
B. Hippocampus
C. Habenula
D. Olfactory bulb
E. Mammillary body

34.

The local anesthetic lidocaine provides analgesia through the blockade of

A. Na$^+$ channels
B. Cl$^-$ channels
C. K$^+$ channels
D. Opioid receptors

35.

The specificity of test X to detect disease Y is

	Disease Y present	Disease Y absent
Test X +	70	25
Test X −	40	55

A. 63.64%
B. 73.68%
C. 68.75%
D. 57.9%

36.

During an endoscopic third ventriculostomy (*arrow*), the mammillary bodies are represented by number

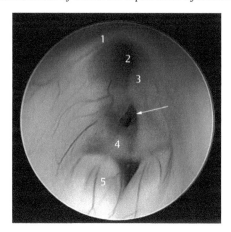

A. 1
B. 2
C. 3
D. 4
E. 5

37.

All of the following are true about the embryonic basal plate, *except* that

A. It connects to the alar plate through the sulcus limitans.
B. It surrounds the ventral part of the ependymal canal.
C. It gives origin to the anterior horn cells of the spinal cord.
D. Cells belong to the mantle zone of the neural tube.
E. It develops at the 15-day embryo.

38.

The inferior cerebellar peduncle carries all of the following, *except*

A. Juxtarestiform body
B. Pontocerebellar fibers
C. Ipsilateral dorsal spinocerebellar tract
D. Cerebello-olivary tract
E. External arcuate fibers

39.

Antidiuretic hormone (ADH) is released from the posterior pituitary, and is synthesized in the

A. Septal nuclei
B. Tuberal nuclei
C. Anterior pituitary
D. Supraoptic nucleus
E. Arcuate nuclei

40.

The stria terminalis connects the amygdala to the

A. Lateral hypothalamus
B. Mammillary bodies
C. Entorhinal cortex
D. Hippocampus
E. Cingulate gyrus

41.

Clopidogrel (Plavix)

A. Inhibits cyclooxygenase 1 (COX-1)
B. Inhibits cyclooxygenase 2 (COX-2)
C. Inhibits ADP-dependent platelet aggregation
D. Prevents thromboxane formation
E. Activates glycoprotein GP IIb/IIIa

42.

The marginal limb of the cingulate sulcus separates the

A. Superior frontal gyrus from the cingulate gyrus
B. Cingulate gyrus from the corpus callosum
C. Superior frontal gyrus from the paracentral lobule
D. Paracentral lobule from the precuneus
E. Precuneus from the cuneus

43.

Which cerebellar nucleus has mostly neocortical projections?

A. Dentate
B. Globose
C. Emboliform
D. Fastigial

44.

The collateral sulcus separates the

A. Precuneus from the cuneus
B. Cuneus from the lingual gyrus
C. Middle temporal gyrus from the inferior temporal gyrus
D. Inferior temporal gyrus from the fusiform gyrus
E. Fusiform gyrus from the parahippocampal gyrus

45.

The best treatment of mercury (Hg) toxicity is

A. British Anti-Lewisite (BAL)
B. 2,3 Dimercapto-1-Propanesulfonate (DMPS)
C. Desferrioxamine
D. Levodopa (L-DOPA)
E. Thiamine

46.

Posterior interosseous nerve (PIN) palsy causes

A. Ulnar deviation with wrist extension
B. Finger drop
C. Paralysis of the interossei
D. Paralysis of the extensor carpi radialis longus
E. Paralysis of the brachioradialis

47.

The nucleus solitarius receives all of the following, *except*

A. Special visceral afferents
B. Fibers from the facial n through the chorda tympani n
C. Fibers from the vestibulocochlear n
D. Fibers from the glossopharyngeal n
E. Fibers from the vagus n

48.

Peroneal n palsy causes all of the following, *except*

A. Loss of sensation in the first web space
B. Paralysis of the tibialis anterior
C. Paralysis of the extensor pollicis longus
D. Paralysis of the tibialis posterior
E. Paralysis of the extensor digitorum longus

49.

A 44-year-old female is being worked-up for headaches. The vessel indicated by *arrows* on the following angiogram and MRI is

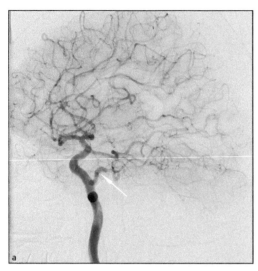

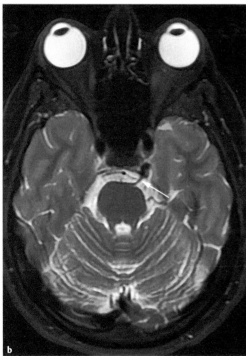

A. Anterior choroidal a

B. Normal PCOM

C. Fetal PCOM

D. Persistent trigeminal a

E. Persistent otic a

50.

The stria medullaris connects the septal nuclei to the

A. Habenula

B. Hypothalamus

C. Hippocampus

D. Interpeduncular nuclei

E. Amygdala

51.

Melanocytes are neural crest derivatives found in high concentration in the

A. Dura mater

B. Leptomeninges

C. Gray matter

D. White matter

E. Ventricular lining

52.

Concerning skeletal muscles, type I fibers have all of the following features, *except*

A. Slow twitch

B. High resistance to fatigue

C. High capillary density

D. Activity during low-intensity endurance exercises

E. Reliance on anaerobic glycolysis

53.

Dabigatran (Pradaxa) is an oral anticoagulant that exerts its function through inhibition of

A. Factor Xa

B. Thrombin

C. Factor VIIIa

D. Factor Va

E. Glycoprotein IIb/IIIa

54.

Isoniazid (INH) is used for treatment of tuberculosis. One of the main side effects is peripheral neuropathy. This can be prevented by supplementing patients with

A. Vitamin A

B. Vitamin B1 (thiamine)

C. Vitamin B6 (pyridoxine)

D. Vitamin B12 (cyanocobalamin)

E. Vitamin C

55.
The main treatment of Wernicke's encephalopathy includes

A.   Vitamin B1 (thiamine)
B.   Vitamin B6 (pyridoxine)
C.   Vitamin B12 (cyanocobalamin)
D.   Vitamin C
E.   Vitamin D

56.
Which of the following drugs correspond with Succinylcholine?

A.   Ganglionic blocker
B.   Neuromuscular blocker
C.   Sympathomimetic
D.   Parasympathomimetic
E.   Alpha adrenergic blocker

57.
Which of the following drugs correspond with Pilocarpine?

A.   Ganglionic blocker
B.   Neuromuscular blocker
C.   Sympathomimetic
D.   Parasympathomimetic
E.   Alpha adrenergic blocker

58.
Which of the following drugs correspond with Prazosin?

A.   Ganglionic blocker
B.   Neuromuscular blocker
C.   Sympathomimetic
D.   Parasympathomimetic
E.   Alpha adrenergic blocker

59.
Which of the following drugs correspond with Amphetamine?

A.   Ganglionic blocker
B.   Neuromuscular blocker
C.   Sympathomimetic
D.   Parasympathomimetic
E.   Alpha adrenergic blocker

60.
Which of the following drugs correspond with Pentolinium?

A.   Ganglionic blocker
B.   Neuromuscular blocker
C.   Sympathomimetic
D.   Parasympathomimetic
E.   Alpha adrenergic blocker

12 Answer Key 6

1.

E Phenylephrine (Neosynephrine)

Phenylephrine (Neosynephrine) is predominantly α_1 stimulant, isoproterenol β, dobutamine β_1, NE α_1 α_2 β_1, epinephrine α_1 α_2 β_1 β_2, and dopamine α_1 α_2 β_1 β_2 Dopa (**Table 33**).

Further Reading: Bangash MN, Kong ML, Pearse RM. Use of inotropes and vasopressor agents in critically ill patients. *Br J Pharmacol.* 2012 Apr;165(7):2015–2033

2.

C Wrist drop

In this location above the elbow, the only large mixed n on the lateral side of the arm is the radial n after it exits the spiral groove. Injury in this location causes wrist drop and spares the triceps. The lateral antebrachial cutaneous n is also close by, but it is purely sensory. The median n is anteromedial and can cause Benediction hand. The ulnar n is posteromedial and can cause Froment's sign and ulnar claw hand. Inability to make the OK sign is caused by injury to the AIN, which is deep in the anterior forearm.

3.

A Thiopental

Thiopental, etomidate, and fentanyl decrease cerebral blood flow. Nitrous oxide, isoflurane, ketamine, enflurane, and halothane increase cerebral blood flow (***Nike Halo***).

4.

C 80 mL/kg

Total blood volume in premature babies 90–100 mL/kg, full term 80 mL/kg, 1 month to 1 year 75 mL/kg, >1 year to adult 70 mL/kg.

5.

B Uric acid

Lasix (furosemide) is a **L**oop diuretic and increases serum GU**L**: glucose, uric acid, and lipids. It decreases K, Ca, Mg, Cl, platelets, and granulocytes. It can lead to hypochloremic alkalosis.

6.

B 150 mL

The normal adult CSF volume is 150 mL, of which 30 mL are intraventricular, 40 mL are in the spinal subarachnoid space, and 80 mL are in the

cranial subarachnoid space. The body produces 3 times the CSF volume per day (450 mL).

7.

A Medial

When targeting STN for Parkinson's disease, if the DBS electrode is too:

- Medial → III n → diplopia, ipsilateral eye adduction.
- Lateral and anterior → internal capsule → contralateral contractions, contralateral gaze deviation.
- Posterior → medial lemniscus → contralateral paresthesias.
- Deep (ventral) → substantia nigra → fear, depression.

8.

B 50 mL/100 g/min

The normal cerebral blood flow is 50 mL/100 g/min, with higher flow in the gray matter than in the white matter. In the ischemic penumbra, it is 8–23 mL/100 g/min. The normal oxygen consumption is 3.5 mL/100 g/min.

9.

B 3

1, Septal v; 2, Thalamostriate v; 3, Internal cerebral v; 4, Basal v of Rosenthal; 5, V of Galen; 6, Straight sinus; 7, Inferior sagittal sinus (**Fig. 5**).

10.

D Deep

When targeting GPi with DBS for Parkinson's disease or dystonia, if the electrode is too:

- Medial and posterior → internal capsule → contralateral contractions.
- Deep → optic tract → phosphenes (flashes of light) in the contralateral visual field.
- Lateral and anterior → GPe, putamen → no effect.

11.

E Diarrhea

The anion gap (AG) is the difference between the primary measured cations (Na^+ and K^+) and the primary measured anions (Cl^- and HCO_3^-). AG = Na^+ – (Cl^- + HCO_3^-) [sometimes excluding potassium]. Normally, it is 3–10 mEq/L (although traditionally considered 12 mEq/L based on older studies). High anion gap acidosis occurs with accumulation of non-measurable anions (e.g., β-hydroxybutarate, acetoacetate, and lactate). This occurs with **MUD PILES**: methanol, uremia, diabetic ketoacidosis, paracetamol, isoniazid, lactic acidosis, ethylene glycol, and salicylates. Also seen in alcoholic keto-acidosis, starvation, and rhabdomyolysis. In cases of diarrhea the drop in HCO_3^- is matched by an increase in Cl^-, so the anion gap is normal.

12.

E 7

1, Dentate gyrus; 2, Cornu Ammonis (hip-pocampus); 3, subiculum; 4, entorhinal cortex; 5, optic tract; 6, temporal horn of lateral ventri-cle; 7, fimbria of fornix; 8, tail of caudate nucleus; 9, alveus; 10, choroid plexus.

13.

A Benzodiazepines

Benzodiazepines, Bactrim, and cimetidine are liver inhibitors that increase the effect of Couma-din with increased risk of bleeding. Barbiturates, rifampicin, and carbamazepine stimulate liver microsomal enzymes, and therefore increase the degradation of warfarin (Coumadin). Cholestyr-amine inhibits gastric absorption of Coumadin.

14.

C Abductor pollicis brevis

The abductor pollicis brevis (APB) is a thenar muscle and is therefore supplied by the median n. The remaining muscles are supplied by the ulnar n.

15.

A Medially

Contralateral gaze deviation during DBS of STN reflects irritation of the internal capsule, which is lateral (and anterior) to STN. The lead should be moved medially. This is not to be confused with irritation of the nucleus of cranial n III, which is medial and causes adduction of the ipsilateral eye.

16.

D 80%

The positive predictive value defines how many subjects actually have the disease out of all who tested positive. In this case $80/(80 + 20) = 80\%$. The negative predictive value reflects how many did not have the disease out of all who tested negative. In this case, 65%.

17.

C Platelets

DIC can occur in conditions like septicemia, and it causes increased clotting, fibrinolysis, and bleeding. There is increased PT, PTT, INR, FDPs, and D-dimers, together with low platelets.

18.

A Gamma-aminobutyric acid (GABA)

The thalamic fasciculus (FFH1) is formed by the lenticular fasciculus (FFH2) and the ansa lenticu-laris. It projects from the GPi to the thalamus using GABA. It also carries dentate nucleus projections to the thalamus (**Fig. 7**).

19.

A Anterior nuclear group (ANG)

The ANG of the thalamus receives input from the fornix and the mamillothalamic tract, and it projects to the cingulate gyrus (**Fig. 8**).

20.

B Sodium nitroprusside (Nipride)

Nipride is a vasodilator used to treat severe hypertension. It releases cyanide into the blood stream and can cause impaired oxygen use. Treat-ment: sodium thiosulfate.

21.

D 4

1, Suprascapular n; 2, musculocutaneous n; 3, median n; 4, ulnar n; 5, radial n; 6, thoracodorsal n; 7, long thoracic n.

22.

E General visceral efferents

The Edinger–Westphal nucleus provides the parasympathetic component of the oculomotor n (III) (general visceral efferent). The general somatic efferents arise from the central nucleus supplying levator palpebrae superioris bilaterally, medial nucleus supplying contralateral superior rectus, and lateral nucleus supplying ipsilateral inferior rectus, inferior oblique, and medial rectus (**Fig. 14**).

23.

A Fastigial

The uncinate fasciculus in the cerebellum con-nects the fastigial nuclei to the contralateral ves-tibular nuclei and travels around the superior cerebellar peduncle, while the juxtarestiform body connects the fastigial nuclei to the ipsilateral vestibular nuclei and travels in the inferior cerebellar peduncle (**Fig. 11**). Not to be confused with the cerebral uncinate fasciculus that connects the orbito-frontal gyri to the anterior temporal lobe.

24.

D Nucleus interpositus
Palatal myoclonus manifests as rhythmic contraction of the soft palate. The jerky movement can cause a clicking sound and is not interrupted by sleep or coma. It is caused by disruption of the Guillain–Mollaret triangle composed of the red nucleus in midbrain, the inferior olivary nucleus in the medulla oblongata, and the contralateral dentate nucleus in the cerebellum.

25.

C VIII
Vitamin K–dependent clotting factors are prothrombin (II), VII, IX, X, and proteins C, S, and Z.

26.

D **It sends efferents in the contralateral dorsal spinocerebellar tract.**
The dorsal spinocerebellar tract travels ipsilaterally through the inferior cerebellar peduncle, while the ventral spinocerebellar tract travels predominantly contralaterally through the superior cerebellar peduncle (**Figs. 11 and 15**).

27.

A Norepinephrine
The locus ceruleus uses NE as neurotransmitter and is responsible for REM sleep (**Figs. 7 and 31**).

28.

A Beta blockers
Beta blockers are harmful to patients with asthma because they cause bronchospasm. Salbutamol is a β_2 agonist and causes bronchodilation. Ipratropium is an anticholinergic (parasympatholytic) bronchodilator. Theophylline and corticosteroids (preferred) are anti-inflammatories.

29.

D Decreased dead space
PEEP increases the dead space by collapsing pulmonary capillaries and to a lesser extent by decreasing cardiac output. It can cause barotrauma. Its main benefit is recruiting collapsed alveoli, thus decreasing the shunt effect.

30.

C Cranial n IV
Structures entering the orbit outside the annulus of Zinn: LFT: lacrimal and frontal branches of V_1, and trochlear n + superior ophthalmic v.

31.

B Binding g-aminobutyric acid type A ($GABA_A$) receptor
Isoflurane and enflurane are $GABA_A$ and glycine stimulants. Lidocaine is a Na^+ channel blocker, fentanyl an opioid agonist, and ketamine an NMDA antagonist (**Table 31**).

32.

B Lateral
Dysarthria and muscle contractions are related to stimulation of the internal capsule which is lateral to the thalamus. Dysarthria could also occur with bilateral Vim stimulation.

33.

A Hypothalamus
The medial forebrain bundle connects the septal nuclei to the hypothalamus. The septal nuclei connect to the habenula through the stria medullaris, to the amygdala through the stria terminalis, and to the hippocampus through the fornix (**Figs. 9 and 10**).

34.

A Na^+ channels
Lidocaine decreases conductance by blocking Na^+ channels. Fentanyl stimulates opioid receptors. Isoflurane, enflurane, etomidate, and thiopental stimulate $GABA_A$, thereby increasing Cl^- influx (**Table 31**).

35.

C 68.8%
Sensitivity marks how often the test is positive when the patient has the disease. In this case 70/(70 + 40) = 63.64%. Specificity indicates how often the test is negative when the disease is absent. In this case 55/(25 + 55) = 68.75%. Prevalence tells how many people had the disease out of all of the people tested (whether positive or negative). In this case (70 + 40)/(70 + 40 + 25 + 55) = 57.89% (rounded 57.9%).

36.

E 5

1, Optic chiasm; 2, pituitary infundibulum; 3, median eminence; 4, tuber cinereum (site for ETV: endoscopic third ventriculostomy); 5, mammillary bodies (see also **Fig. 23B**).

37.

E It develops at the 15-day embryo.

The basal plate contains primarily motor neurons, while the alar plate is predominantly sensory. They are separated by the sulcus limitans. This is a postneurulation event (>22 days). With the development of the fourth ventricle, the alar plates are moved posterolaterally (pontine flexure) (**Fig. 12**).

38.

B Pontocerebellar fibers

The pontocerebellar fibers travel in the middle cerebellar peduncle.

39.

D Supraoptic nucleus

ADH (vas**op**ressin) is synthesized in the supra**op**tic nucleus, while oxytocin is predominantly synthesized in the paraventricular nucleus. Both are secreted by the posterior pituitary gland (neurohypophysis).

40.

A Lateral hypothalamus

The stria terminalis connects the amygdala to the lateral hypothalamus and septal nuclei (**Figs. 9 and 10**).

41.

C Inhibits ADP-dependent platelet aggregation

Clopidogrel (Plavix) inhibits the binding of ADP to P2Y12 receptor on platelets → inhibits activation of glycoprotein GP IIb/IIIa → inhibits platelet aggregation. Aspirin (ASA) → inhibits cyclo-oxygenase (COX-1 and COX-2) in platelets → inhibits platelet-dependent thromboxane formation → inhibits platelet aggregation. ReoPro (abciximab) and Integrilin (eptifibatide) are glycoprotein GP IIb/IIIa inhibitors → inhibit platelet aggregation (**Fig. 32**).

42.

D Paracentral lobule from the precuneus

The cingulate sulcus separates the cingulate gyrus from the superior frontal gyrus, while its marginal limb separates the paracentral lobule from the precuneus. The parieto-occipital sulcus separates the precuneus from the cuneus. The calcarine sulcus separates the cuneus from the lingual gyrus. The callosal sulcus separates the corpus callosum from the cingulate gyrus (**Fig. 2**).

43.

A Dentate

The dentate nucleus is part of the neocerebellum, the globose and emboliform nuclei belong to the paleocerebellum, and the fastigial nucleus represents the archicerebellum.

44.

E Fusiform gyrus from the parahippocampal gyrus

The superior temporal sulcus separates superior (T1) from middle temporal gyri (T2). The middle temporal sulcus separates middle (T2) from inferior temporal gyri (T3). The occipitotemporal sulcus separates inferior temporal (T3) from fusiform (T4) gyri. The collateral sulcus separates fusiform (occipitotemporal) (T4) from parahippocampal (T5) gyri. The parieto-occipital sulcus separates the precuneus from the cuneus. The calcarine sulcus separates the cuneus from the lingual gyrus (**Figs. 1 and 2**).

45.

B 2,3 Dimercapto-1-Propanesulfonate (DMPS

Dimercaprol (British Anti-Lewisite, BAL) is used as a chelating agent in arsenic poisoning, while penicillamine, DMPS, and DMSA (dimercaptosuccinic acid) are effective in mercury toxicity. BAL, penicillamine, EDTA (ethylene diamine tetraacetic acid), and DMSA are used for lead poisoning, while desferrioxamine is used to treat iron and aluminium toxicities. Manganese toxicity affects basal ganglia (GPi) and is treated by L-DOPA, and ethanol toxicity is treated by thiamine (**Table 30**).

46.

B Finger drop

The PIN passes under the edge of the supinator (Fröhse arcade). Paralysis leads to finger drop and radial deviation with wrist extension due to the intact extensor carpi radialis longus and brevis while the extensor carpi ulnaris is paralyzed.

47.

C Fibers from the vestibulocochlear n

The nucleus solitarius receives special visceral afferents of taste from VII (anterior 2/3 of tongue),

IX (posterior 1/3 of tongue), and X (epiglottis, vallecula), and general visceral afferents from the salivary glands, carotid body, chest, and abdomen (**Fig. 14**).

48.

D Paralysis of the tibialis posterior

The tibialis posterior is supplied by the tibial n and causes intact inversion in the setting of a peroneal n palsy.

49.

D Persistent trigeminal a

The patient has a persistent trigeminal a that connects the precavernous ICA to the basilar a. Note that the patient also has a fetal PCOM right above (more distally) and almost parallel to the vessel with the *arrow*.

50.

A Habenula

The septal nuclei connect to the habenula through the stria medullaris, to the hypothalamus through the medial forebrain bundle, to the amygdala through the stria terminalis, and to the hippocampus through the fornix (**Figs. 9** and **10**).

51.

B Leptomeninges

Melanocytes are found in the leptomeninges and can cause primary melanocytic tumors of the CNS. They can be focal or diffuse.

52.

E Reliance on anaerobic glycolysis

Type I fibers have a high mitochondrial content, rely more on oxidative metabolism, and produce little lactic acid (**Table 4**).

53.

B Thrombin

Pradaxa is an oral thrombin inhibitor. PCC (Kcentra, prothrombin complex concentrate) can be used for reversal in bleeding emergencies. Idarucizumab (Praxbind) is an antibody that can bind and reverse Pradaxa. Lepirudin and argatroban are IV thrombin inhibitors. Xarelto, Eliquis, Lovenox, and Arixtra are all factor Xa inhibitors. Protein C

inhibits Va and VIIIa. Integrilin and ReoPro inhibit GP IIb/IIIa, thus inhibiting platelet aggregation (**Fig. 32**).

54.

C Vitamin B6 (pyridoxine)

INH creates a state of pyridoxine (vitamin B6) deficiency, causing peripheral neuropathy.

55.

A Vitamin B1 (thiamine)

IV thiamine is used to treat Wernicke's encephalopathy. It is an acute complication of alcohol abuse manifested by ataxia, nystagmus, confusion, dysconjugate gaze, lateral rectus palsy, hypothermia, hypotension, coma, and death (17%) (**Table 30**).

56.

B Neuromuscular blocker

Succinylcholine is a depolarizing neuromuscular blocker (**Fig 25**). In patients with ryanodine receptor mutation, it can cause malignant hyperthermia (**Table 13**).

57.

D Parasympathomimetic

Pilocarpine is a parasympathomimetic stimulating muscarinic acetylcholine receptor. It is used to treat dry mouth and glaucoma (**Fig. 25**).

58.

E Alpha adrenergic blocker

Prazosin is an α_1 adrenergic blocker used to treat arterial hypertension (**Fig. 25**).

59.

C Sympathomimetic

Amphetamine stimulates the release of norepinephrine from postganglionic sympathetic nerve endings (**Fig. 25**). It is used to treat ADHD (attention deficit hyperactivity disorder).

60.

A Ganglionic blocker

Pentolinium is a ganglionic blocker: antagonist to nicotinic acetylcholine receptors in autonomic ganglia. It is used to treat hypertension (**Fig. 25**).

13 Test 7—Pathology, Radiology, and Neurology

1.

While preparing for surgery for the following posterior fossa tumor, the surgeon and anesthesiologist should be aware of

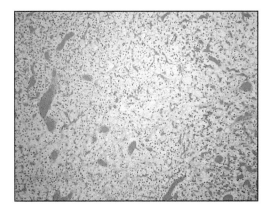

A. Risk of hypertension
B. Risk of hematuria
C. Pressure points due to associated cutaneous neurofibromas
D. Difficult intubation due to sphenoid dysplasia
E. Risk of seizures

2.

When the following tumor is associated with meningiomas and basal cell nevus syndrome, the most likely abnormality occurs on which chromosome?

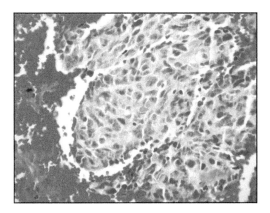

A. 3
B. 5
C. 9
D. 11
E. 22

3.

The following applies to malignant hyperthermia, *except*

A. Autosomal dominant inheritance
B. Caused by a defect in porphobilinogen deaminase
C. Elevated creatine kinase (CK)
D. Hyperkalemia
E. Treated with dantrolene

4.

The following tumor was removed from the lateral ventricle of an adult male and was positive for synaptophysin. What is the diagnosis?

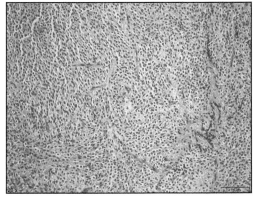

A. Oligodendroglioma
B. Medulloblastoma
C. Choroid plexus papilloma
D. Subependymoma
E. Central neurocytoma

5.

Neurofibrillary tangles and neuritic plaques are characteristic of which disease?

A. Alzheimer's
B. Pick's
C. Wilson's
D. Parkinson's
E. Hallervorden–Spatz

6.

A unilateral headache in a young adult male associated with rhinorrhea, lacrimation, and conjunctival injection is characteristic of

A.   Classic migraine
B.   Common migraine
C.   Migraine variant
D.   Cluster headache
E.   Temporal arteritis

7.

Which of the following vasculitides affects large and medium-sized vessels and causes interstitial keratitis, Ménière's symptoms, hearing loss, and cavernous sinus thrombosis?

A.   Cogan's syndrome
B.   Behçet's disease
C.   Buerger's disease
D.   Wegener's granulomatosis
E.   Takayasu's arteritis

8.

Which of the following does *not* apply to the tumor depicted below?

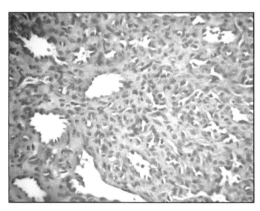

A.   Male predominance
B.   Mostly supratentorial
C.   High recurrence rate
D.   Never metastasizes
E.   Excessive bleeding in surgery

9.

Gargoyle face, thick meninges, deafness, and hepatosplenomegaly are found in which mucopolysaccharidose?

A.   Hunter's syndrome
B.   Hurler's disease
C.   Sanfilippo's syndrome
D.   Morquio's syndrome
E.   Maroteaux–Lamy syndrome

10.

A 74-year-old female presents with a 2-week history of speech impairment and right upper extremity weakness. She subsequently worsened neurologically and died. Autopsy findings are below. The most likely diagnosis is

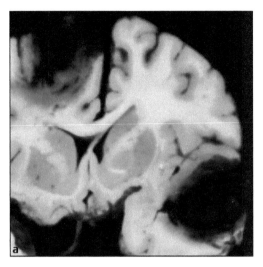

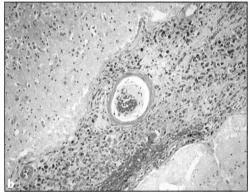

A.   Left MCA aneurysm
B.   Pericallosal artery aneurysm
C.   Hypertensive bleed
D.   Amyloid angiopathy
E.   Arterio-venous malformation

11.

The following depicted abnormality is caused by a disorder of

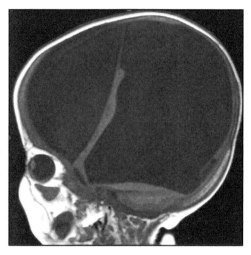

A.   Primary neurulation
B.   Secondary neurulation
C.   Ventral induction
D.   Migration

12.

A 48-year-old male presents with stupor and right-sided hemiplegia. The patient's grade is

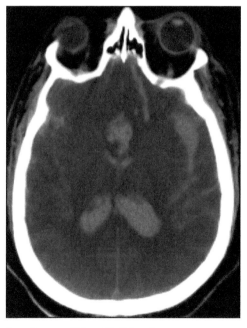

A.   Hunt and Hess III, Fisher 3
B.   Hunt and Hess IV, Fisher 4
C.   Hunt and Hess III, Fisher 4
D.   Hunt and Hess IV, Fisher 3
E.   Hunt and Hess V, Fisher 4

13.

A cerebral angiogram is performed, revealing an aneurysm of

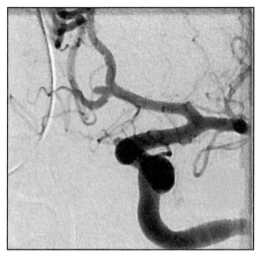

A.   ACOM
B.   MCA
C.   Pericallosal artery
D.   PCOM
E.   Paraclinoid

14.

A cherry-red spot in the macula is found in all of the following lysosomal storage diseases, *except*

A.   GM1 gangliosidosis
B.   Sandhoff's disease
C.   Tay–Sachs disease
D.   Gaucher's disease
E.   Niemann–Pick's disease

15.

A defect in hypoxanthine guanine phospho-ribosyl transferase (HGPRT) causes

A.   Lesch–Nyhan disease
B.   Menke's kinky hair disease
C.   Lowe's syndrome
D.   Zellweger's syndrome
E.   Leigh's disease

16.

Collet–Sicard syndrome involves all of the following cranial nerves, *except*

A.   VII
B.   IX
C.   X
D.   XI
E.   XII

17.

The tumor depicted in the following figure can be associated with all of the following, *except*

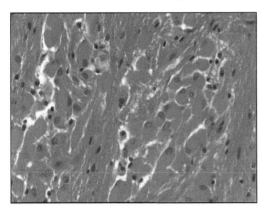

A. Seizures
B. Posterior fossa location
C. Subungal fibroma (Koenen tumor)
D. Adenoma sebaceum (facial angiofibroma)
E. Cardiac rhabdomyoma

18.

The lesion depicted in the following T1-weighted MRI without contrast is most likely a(n)

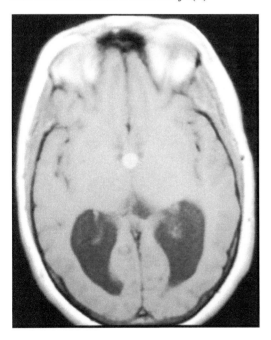

A. Subependymoma
B. Choroid plexus papilloma
C. Colloid cyst
D. Ependymoma
E. Subependymal giant cell astrocytoma (SEGA)

19.

The abnormality depicted in this MRI is caused by a congenital anomaly that occurs at which gestational age?

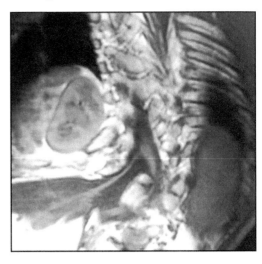

A. 3–4 weeks
B. 4–5 weeks
C. 5–10 weeks
D. 2–5 months
E. After 5 months

20.

The following tumor was most likely removed from

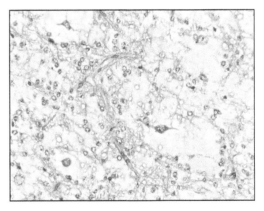

A. The temporal lobe of a child with seizures
B. The cerebellum of a child
C. The fourth ventricle in an adult
D. The lateral ventricle at the foramen of Monro
E. The frontal lobe of an adult with seizures

21.

The following is an axial CT scan at T10 performed on a 13-year-old boy with back pain that responds well to Aspirin. The most likely diagnosis is

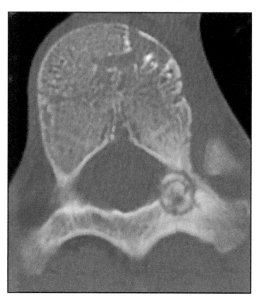

A. Osteoblastoma
B. Osteosarcoma
C. Chondrosarcoma
D. Paget's disease
E. Osteoid osteoma

22.

Hearing loss, visual loss, peripheral neuropathy, and impaired microtubule function are observed with which of the following toxicities?

A. Arsenic
B. Lead
C. Mercury
D. Cisplatin
E. Methotrexate

23.

The following are the histological findings when this posterior fossa mass was removed. What is the diagnosis?

A. Pilocytic astrocytoma
B. Hemangioblastoma
C. Blastomycosis
D. Ependymoma
E. Medulloblastoma

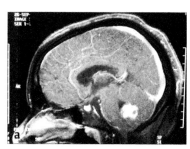
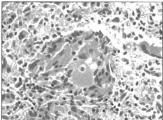
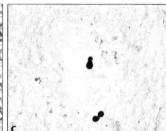

24.

Lisch nodules are a feature of which phacomatosis?

A.   Neurofibromatosis type 1
B.   Neurofibromatosis type 2
C.   Tuberous sclerosis
D.   Von Hippel–Lindau disease
E.   Sturge–Weber syndrome

25.

The first line of treatment in status epilepticus is

A.   Barbiturates
B.   Benzodiazepines
C.   Phenytoin
D.   Carbamazepine
E.   Propofol

26.

Synaptophysin is usually positive in

A.   Central neurocytoma
B.   Craniopharyngioma
C.   Meningioma
D.   Oligodendroglioma
E.   Germinoma

27.

The brain biopsy depicted below is from an AIDS (acquired immune deficiency syndrome) patient with multiple brain lesions. The diagnosis is

A.   Lymphoma
B.   Toxoplasmosis
C.   Metastasis
D.   Cryptococcal meningitis
E.   Herpes encephalitis

28.

Peripheral neuropathy with basophilic stippling of red blood corpuscles is characteristic of which toxicity?

A.   Methanol
B.   Arsenic
C.   Mercury
D.   Manganese
E.   Lead

29.

The following axial T2-weighted MRI at L4–L5 from a patient presenting with left L5 radiculopathy is mostly consistent with

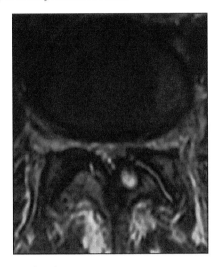

A.   Cystic schwannoma
B.   Meningioma
C.   Tarlov cyst
D.   Synovial cyst
E.   Metastasis

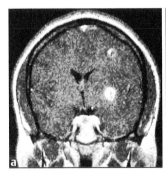
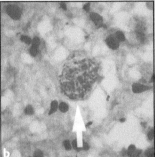
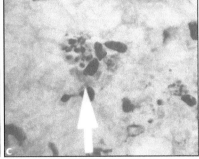

30.

Amyotrophic lateral sclerosis (ALS) is associated with abnormality of

A. Dystrophin
B. Ryanodine receptor
C. Cu/Zn superoxide dismutase
D. Phytanic acid oxidase
E. Phenylalanine hydroxylase

31.

During brainstem auditory evoked responses (BAER), the wave that corresponds to the lateral lemniscus is number

A. II
B. III
C. IV
D. V
E. VI

32.

Fibrillation potential can be observed on EMG in the following cases, *except*

A. Motor cortex stroke
B. Amyotrophic lateral sclerosis
C. Poliomyelitis
D. Radiculopathy
E. Peripheral neuropathy

33.

Opsoclonus–myoclonus can occur in breast cancer and correlate with which of the following antibodies?

A. Anti-Ri
B. Anti-Hu
C. Anti-Tr
D. Anti-Yo
E. Anti-Jo

34.

Hypsarrhythmias observed on EEG are characteristics of

A. Juvenile myoclonic epilepsy (JME)
B. Infantile spasms (West syndrome)
C. Benign focal epilepsy of childhood
D. Petit mal (absence) epilepsy
E. Grand mal epilepsy

35.

The structure shown below (*arrow*) is typically seen in which tumor?

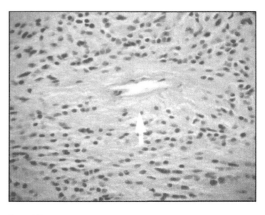

A. Pineocytoma
B. Pineoblastoma
C. Medulloblastoma
D. Ependymoma
E. Neuroblastoma

36.

In multiple endocrine neoplasia type 1 (MEN1), pituitary adenomas are associated with parathyroid and pancreatic islet tumors. This is typically due to an abnormality on which chromosome?

A. 3
B. 5
C. 9
D. 11
E. 17

37.

All of the following characterize Cowden's disease, *except*

A. Abnormality in chromosome 9
B. Lhermitte–Duclos disease
C. Breast cancer
D. Uterine cancer
E. Thyroid cancer

38.

When atrophy of the shoulder and pelvic girdles is associated with calf pseudohypertrophy and a positive Gower's test, the most likely diagnosis is

A. Mitochondrial myopathy
B. Limb–girdle muscular dystrophy
C. Kearns–Sayre syndrome
D. Emery–Dreifuss muscular dystrophy
E. Duchenne's muscular dystrophy

39.

On immunohistochemistry, the tumor depicted below is typically positive for

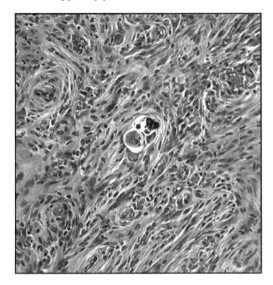

A. Epithelial membrane antigen (EMA)
B. Glial fibrillary acid protein (GFAP)
C. S100
D. Transthyretin
E. Cytokeratin

40.

A 38-year-old female is being worked up for acute onset of headaches and vertigo. The vessel shown by the *arrow* on her DSA is

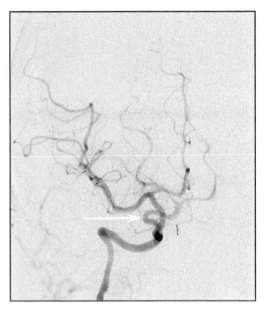

A. PCOM
B. Anterior choroidal a
C. Persistent trigeminal a
D. Hypoglossal a
E. Proatlantal a

41.

The main finding on the CT scan shown below is

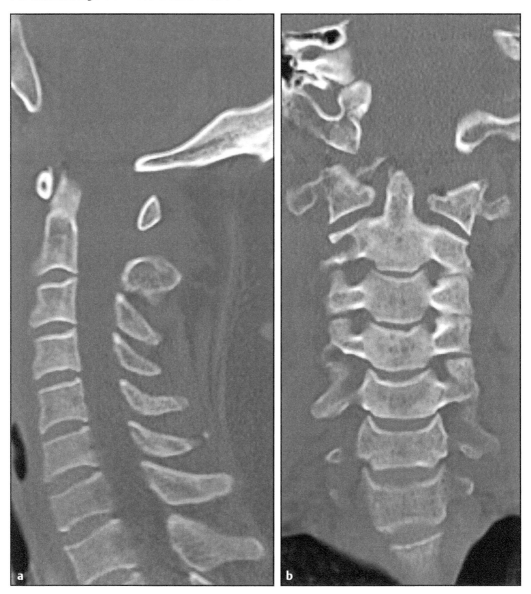

A.   C1–C2 subluxation
B.   Atlanto-occipital dislocation (AOD)
C.   Type II dens fracture
D.   Jefferson fracture
E.   Rupture of the transverse ligament of atlas

42.

The following pathological findings from a clival tumor are consistent with

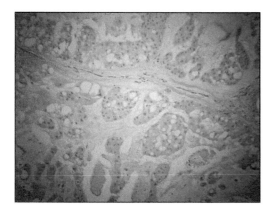

A. Meningioma
B. Osteosarcoma
C. Chordoma
D. Chondrosarcoma
E. Metastasis

43.

The following T1-weighted MRI images with contrast and diffusion are consistent with the diagnosis of

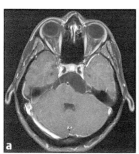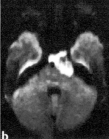

A. Dermoid tumor
B. Epidermoid tumor
C. Arachnoid cyst
D. Vestibular schwannoma
E. Meningioma

44.

The vessel causing the blush from the tumor depicted below is the

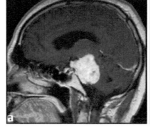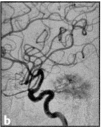

A. A of Bernasconi and Cassinari
B. McConnell's capsular a
C. A of Percheron
D. Inferior hypophyseal a
E. Superior hypophyseal a

45.

The findings in the following picture are typical for

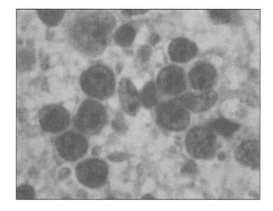

A. Plasmacytoma
B. Central neurocytoma
C. Medulloblastoma
D. Greminoma
E. Primary CNS lymphoma

46.

The following MRI findings are characteristic for

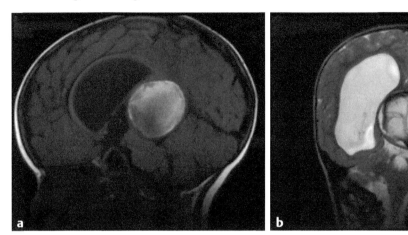

A. Germinoma
B. Teratoma
C. Dermoid cyst
D. Giant thrombosed basilar tip aneurysm
E. Vein of Galen malformation

47.

A 32-year-old female presents with blurring of vision and left arm numbness. MRI findings are consistent with

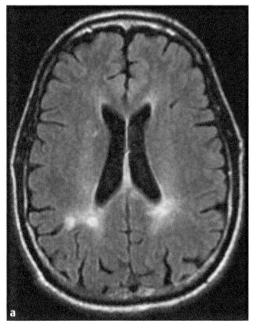

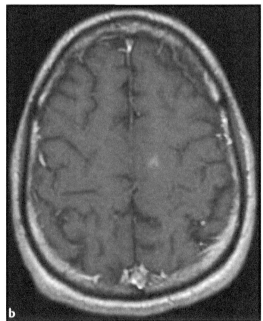

A. Transient ischemic attacks (TIAs)
B. Brain abscesses
C. Hypertension
D. Multiple sclerosis (MS)
E. Gliomatosis cerebri

48.

Macrocephaly is observed with which leukodystrophy?

A. Canavan's disease
B. Krabbe's disease
C. Metachromatic leukodystrophy
D. Adrenoleukodystrophy
E. Pelizaeus–Merzbacher disease

49.

The following MRI findings are more likely to be seen in

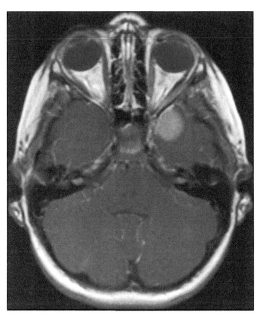

A. Sporadic meningioma
B. Neurofibromatosis type 1
C. Neurofibromatosis type 2
D. Tuberous sclerosis
E. Von Hippel–Lindau disease

50.

The following histological finding is typical for

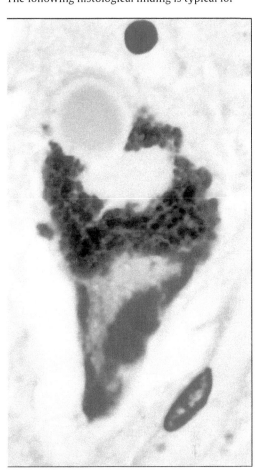

A. Measles
B. Rabies
C. Parkinson's disease
D. Alzheimer's disease
E. Amyotrophic lateral sclerosis

51.

The following CT is from a patient that presents with incomplete spinal cord injury. The most important step that affects the patient's outcome is

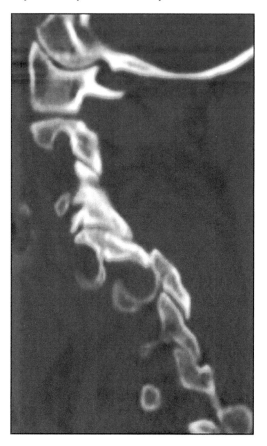

A. MRI
B. Awake reduction with traction
C. ACDF (anterior cervical discectomy and fusion)
D. PCF (posterior cervical fusion)
E. Halo-vest stabilization

52.

The following two MRI findings most likely show

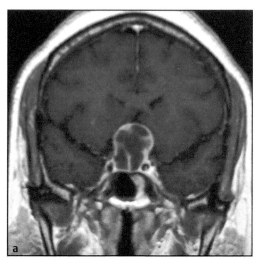

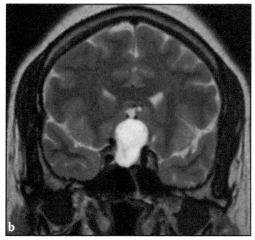

A. Craniopharyngioma
B. Rathke's cleft cyst
C. Pituitary adenoma
D. Lymphocytic hypophysitis
E. Germinoma

53.

The lesion depicted by the following T1-(**a**) and T2-weighted (**b**) MRI pictures most likely represents

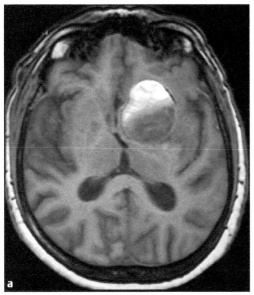

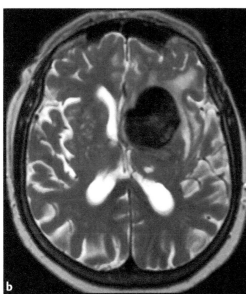

A. Giant thrombosed aneurysm
B. Meningioma
C. Intraparenchymal hematoma
D. Glioblastoma multiforme (GBM)
E. Pleomorphic xanthoastrocytoma (PXA)

54.

All of the following are features of myasthenia gravis, *except*

A. Association with thymomas
B. Extraocular muscle weakness
C. Antibodies to nicotinic acetylcholine receptors
D. Incremental response to repetitive nerve stimulation
E. Treatment with anticholinesterase medications

55.

The following histologic findings are consistent with

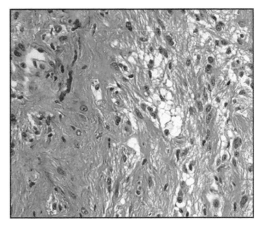

A. Meningioma
B. Fibrillary astrocytoma
C. Glioblastoma multiforme
D. Pleomorphic xanthoastrocytoma (PXA)
E. Pilocytic astrocytoma

56.

Which of the following finds correspond with Measles?

A. Negri bodies
B. Bunina bodies
C. Hirano bodies
D. Lewy bodies
E. Multinucleated cells

57.

Which of the following finds correspond with Rabies?

A. Negri bodies
B. Bunina bodies
C. Hirano bodies
D. Lewy bodies
E. Multinucleated cells

58.

Which of the following finds correspond with Alzheimer's disease?

A. Negri bodies
B. Bunina bodies
C. Hirano bodies
D. Lewy bodies
E. Multinucleated cells

59.

Which of the following finds correspond with Amyotrophic lateral sclerosis (ALS)?

A. Negri bodies
B. Bunina bodies
C. Hirano bodies
D. Lewy bodies
E. Multinucleated cells

60.

Which of the following finds correspond with Parkinson's disease?

A. Negri bodies
B. Bunina bodies
C. Hirano bodies
D. Lewy bodies
E. Multinucleated cells

14 Answer Key 7

1.

A Risk of hypertension

Hemangioblastoma is the most common primary intra-axial tumor in the posterior fossa. Radiologically, it typically appears cystic with an enhancing mural nodule. Histologically, it is characterized by hemorrhage and clear cells (not to be confused with metastatic renal cell carcinoma, which would be positive for EMA). It stains positive for reticulin and vimentin. In 20% of cases, it is associated with von Hippel–Lindau (VHL) disease (chromosome 3). Pheochromocytoma occurs in 10% of cases of VHL and can cause severe hypertension during surgery. Patients should be screened by plasma metanephrine, urinary catecholamines, metanephrine, and VMA (**Table 11**).

2.

C 9

Medulloblastoma, here characterized by large blue nuclei with little cytoplasm molded to each other and Homer–Wright rosettes. When part of Gorlin's syndrome (chromosome 9), it can be associated with meningioma and benign cell nevus syndrome (**Table 11**). In medulloblastomas, *WNT* has the best prognosis and group 3 has the worst. Other types, including sonic hedgehog (SHH) and group 4, have intermediate prognosis.

3.

B Caused by a defect in porphobilinogen deaminase

Malignant hyperthermia is autosomal dominant, on chromosome 19q, is caused by ryanodine receptor mutation, and causes increased Ca^{++} release from sarcoplasmic reticulum, increased CK, hyperkalemia, and myoglobinuria. It occurs with halothane and succinylcholine, and is characterized by fever, rigidity, hyperventilation, tachycardia, dysrhythmia, hypertension, and hypotension. Treatment includes dantrolene. Defect in porphobilinogen deaminase is associated with acute intermittent porphyria, not malignant hyperthermia (**Table 13**).

4.

E Central neurocytoma

Central neurocytomas are intraventricular tumors of young adults. They occur in the region of the foramen of Monro, typically attach to the septum pellucidum, and enhance with contrast (moderate and heterogeneous). Histologically, they are small cells with halos and can be mistaken for oligodendrogliomas. Immunohistochemistry is positive for synaptophysin, and electron microscopy reveals dense-core synaptic vesicles. Subependymomas are common in the fourth ventricle and don't enhance. Histologically, they have a spongy appearance with microcysts.

5.

A Alzheimer's

Alzheimer's disease is characterized by neurofibrillary tangles (tau protein), neuritic plaques (β/α protein amyloid), and Hirano bodies. Pick's disease is characterized by Pick bodies, Parkinson's disease by Lewy bodies, Wilson's disease by Opalski cells, and Hallervorden–Spatz disease by iron deposition in SN and GP (**Table 14**).

6.

D Cluster headache

Cluster headache is a "hypersecretion" headache due to parasympathetic discharge. Classic migraine has aura while common migraine has no aura. Migraine variant has less headache and more neurological deficits. Temporal arteritis is characterized by headache, jaw pain, shoulder pain, loss of vision, thick tender scalp vessels, high ESR, and giant cells on temporal a biopsy. Treat with corticosteroids until the ESR is normal.

7.

A Cogan's syndrome

Cogan's syndrome can manifest by interstitial keratitis, Ménière's symptoms, hearing loss, headaches, peripheral neuropathy, and cavernous sinus thrombosis. Behçet's disease is characterized by orogenital ulcers, arthritis, and uveitis. Buerger's disease (or thromboangiitis obliterans) occurs with tobacco smoking. Wegener's granulomatosis affects respiratory, renal, and intracranial vessels and causes peripheral and cranial neuropathies. Takayasu's arteritis affects the aorta and pulmonary arteries and can cause visual loss (**Table 29**).

8.

D Never metastasizes

Staghorn blood vessels are characteristic of hemangiopericytoma. They also stain positive for reticulin. They are common in middle-age, with slight male preponderance. They tend to recur and can metastasize.

Further Reading: Rutkowski MJ, Sughrue ME, Kane AJ, et al. Predictors of mortality following treatment of intracranial hemangiopericytoma. *J Neurosurg.* 2010 Aug;113(2):333–339

9.

B Hurler's disease

Hurler's disease (mucopolysaccharidose MPS 1H) is an autosomal recessive disease due to α-L-iduronidase deficiency. Features include: Zebra bodies, increased urine heparin and dermatan sulfate, gargoyle face, mental retardation, and hepatosplenomegaly (**Table 12**).

10.

D Amyloid angiopathy

Cerebral amyloid angiopathy characterized by amyloid deposition in the vessel wall replacing the media. The patient is elderly with multifocal intracerebral hemorrhage.

11.

C Ventral induction

MRI reveals alobar holoprosencephaly, which is a disorder of ventral induction that occurs between 5 and 10 weeks (**Table 9**).

12.

B Hunt and Hess IV, Fisher 4

Because of hemiplegia, the patient is Hunt and Hess grade IV (**Table 22**), and with intraventricular blood, the patient is Fisher grade 4 (**Table 23**).

13.

A ACOM

The angiogram reveals an ACOM aneurysm (*arrow*).

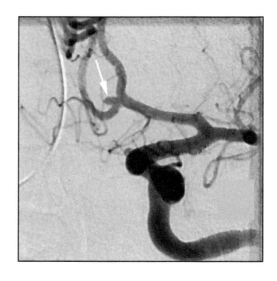

14.

D Gaucher's disease

A cherry-red spot in the macula is characteristic of GM1 gangliosidosis, Sandhoff's disease, Tay–Sachs disease, and Niemann–Pick disease. Gaucher's disease and Fabry's disease do not have a cherry-red spot in the macula (**Table 12**).

15.

A Lesch–Nyhan disease

Lesch–Nyhan disease is X-linked recessive, caused by a defect in hypoxanthine guanine phospho-ribosyl transferase, and characterized by uric acid accumulation, self-mutilation, and choreoathetosis (**Table 12**).

16.

A VII

Collet–Sicard syndrome is a unilateral lower cranial nerve syndrome. It affects cranial nerves IX–XII. It is caused by skull base lesions close to the jugular foramen, e.g., glomus jugulare tumor or occipital condyle fractures (**Table 15**).

17.

B Posterior fossa location

Subependymal giant cell astrocytoma (SEGA) can be associated with tuberous sclerosis. It is inherited on chromosome 9 or 16 as autosomal dominant (**Table 11**). SEGA occurs in the region of the foramen of Monro and is characterized by large cells with large eccentric nuclei.

18.

C Colloid cyst

Colloid cysts occur in the region of foramen of Monro and are typically hyperdense on a non-contrast head CT, hyperintense on T1 MRI, and hypointense on T2 MRI.

19.

B 4–5 weeks

MRI reveals diastematomyelia, or split spinal cord, which occurs due to abnormal disjunction (secondary neurulation) at 4–5 weeks gestation (**Table 9**).

20.

A The temporal lobe of a child with seizures

Dysembryoplastic neuroepithelial tumor (DNET) typically occurs in the temporal lobe in children and causes seizures. It is characterized by neurons floating in mucinous material, chicken wire vessels, and small oligodendrocyte-like cells.

21.

E Osteoid osteoma

Osteoid osteoma occurs in children, has a target sign on CT, and responds well to NSAIDs.

22.

D Cisplatin

Cisplatin causes peripheral neuropathy, impaired hearing, and vision. Cisplatin attacks tubulin which affects microtubule function. Vincristine and vinblastine impair microtubule function, resulting in axonal peripheral neuropathy. Mercury affects the rough endoplasmic reticulum, thus inhibiting translation and causes peripheral neuropathy (**Table 30, Fig. 29**).

23.

C Blastomycosis

*B*lastomycosis is characterized by *b*udding yeast.

24.

A Neurofibromatosis type 1

Lisch nodules are a major diagnostic criterion for NF1, which is inherited as autosomal dominant on chromosome 17. NF2 is characterized by bilateral vestibular schwannomas, tuberous sclerosis by SEGA, facial angiofibroma and ash leaf spots, and von Hippel–Lindau by hemangioblastomas.

Sturge–Weber features tram-track calcification of blood vessels (on CT) and port-wine stain of the skin of the face (**Table 11**).

25.

B Benzodiazepines

A benzodiazepine (lorazepam [Ativan] 0.1 mg/kg IV, diazepam [Valium] 0.2 mg/kg IV, or midazolam [Versed] 0.2 mg/kg) is the first line of treatment in status epilepticus, in addition to loading with Dilantin.

26.

A Central neurocytoma

Synaptophysin is positive in central neurocytoma (synaptic vesicles are seen on electron microscopy), vi*men*tin and epithelial membrane antigen (*EMA*) in *men*ingiomas, placental alkaline phosphatase in germinoma, and 1p19q deletion in oligodendrogliomas.

27.

B Toxoplasmosis

Toxoplasmosis is a common infection in AIDS patients. Radiologically, a ring-enhancing lesion with a target sign is seen on CT or MRI (a). Histologically, *b*radyzoites are *b*ound in cysts (*b*ags) (b, *arrow*), while tachyzoites are loose (c, *arrow*).

28.

E Lead

Basophilic stippling of red blood corpuscles is characteristic of lead poisoning, mercury causes defective translation and affects the cerebellum, manganese causes neuronal loss in the pallidum and striatum, and arsenic causes Mees' lines (transverse white lines on finger nails) and pancytopenia while methanol causes necrosis of putamen and claustrum, optic disc swelling, and high anion gap acidosis (**Table 30, Figs. 7 and 29**).

29.

D Synovial cyst

Synovial cysts are common at L4-L5 level, usually unilateral, associated with the facet joints, and hyperintense on T2 due to synovial fluid content. Flexion/extension X-rays may demonstrate instability. Tarlov cysts are described in the sacrum. Schwannomas and meningiomas are typically intradural. Metastases are usually associated with the pedicle or vertebral body, not the facet joints.

30.

C Cu/Zn superoxide dismutase

Cu/Zn superoxide dismutase abnormality is associated with ALS, dystrophin with Duchenne, Becker, and limb–girdle muscle dystrophy, ryanodine receptor with malignant hyperthermia, phytanic acid oxidase with Refsum's disease, and phenylalanine hydroxylase with phenylketonuria (**Tables 12 and 13**).

31.

C IV

BAER waves: I, cochlear nerve; II, cochlear nuclei; III, superior olivary nucleus; IV, lateral lemniscus; V, inferior colliculus; VI, medial geniculate body; and VII, auditory radiation (**Fig. 31**).

Further Reading: Guerreiro CA, Ehrenberg BL. Brainstem auditory evoked response: application in neurology. *Arq Neuropsiquiatr.* 1982 Mar;40(1):21–28

32.

A Motor cortex stroke

Fibrillation potential is a spontaneous action potential obtained when a muscle is denervated (lower motor disease, B–E).

Further Reading: Feinberg J. EMG: myths and facts. *HSS J.* 2006 Feb;2(1):19–21

Willmott AD, White C, Dukelow SP. Fibrillation potential onset in peripheral nerve injury. *Muscle Nerve* 2012 Sep;46(3):332–340

33.

A Anti-Ri

Anti-**R**i occurs in b**r**east cancer and causes opsoclonus-myoclonus, anti-H**u** in small cell l**u**ng cancer and lymphoma and causes peripheral ne**u**ropathy, anti-T**r** in Hodgkin's lymphoma and involves the ante**r**ior ho**r**n cells and ce**r**ebellum, anti-Y**o** in **o**varian cancer and affects the cerebellum, and anti-**J**o in crypt**og**enic fibrosing alveolitis and causes polymyositis (**Table 16**).

34.

B Infantile spasms (West syndrome)

Hypsarrhythmia is characterized by bilateral large slow waves with multifocal spikes on EEG. It occurs in West syndrome (infantile spasms). Treatment includes ACTH (**Table 34, Fig. 31**). Spike-dome waves occur in absence (3 Hz), JME (4–6 Hz), and Lennox–Gastaut (1–2 Hz). Benign focal epilepsy of childhood is characterized by centro-temporal spikes.

35.

D Ependymoma

E**p**endymomas are characterized by **p**seudorosettes that occur around **b**lood vessels. Medulloblastomas have Homer–Wright rosettes (no central vessel or lumen). Pineoblastomas, retinoblastomas, and ependymomas have Flexner–Wintersteiner rosettes (columnar cells with central lumen), while pineocytomas have very large rosettes (**Table 7**).

36.

D 11

MEN **1** (Wermer's syndrome) is inherited as autosomal dominant on chromosome **11** (**Table 11**).

37.

A Abnormality in chromosome 9

Cowden's disease is inherited as autosomal dominant on chromosome 10 (PTEN mutation) (**Table 11**).

Further Reading: Liaw D, Marsh DJ, Li J, et al. Germline mutations of the PTEN gene in Cowden disease, an inherited breast and thyroid cancer syndrome. *Nat Genet.* 1997 May;16(1):64–67

38.

E Duchenne's muscle dystrophy

Duchenne's muscle dystrophy is characterized by atrophy of the shoulder and pelvic girdles, calf pseudohypertrophy and positive Gower's test. There is also congestive heart failure, respiratory infections, and occasionally mental retardation. It is inherited as X-linked recessive. There is decreased dystrophin and increased CK as well as muscle fiber necrosis and regeneration. Treatment includes corticosteroids (**Table 13**).

39.

A Epithelial membrane antigen (EMA)

Meningiomas are positive for **EM**A and vi**men**tin. The photomicrograph shows a meningioma with its characteristic whorls and a calcified psammoma body (*arrow*). GFAP is characteristic of astrocytomas, S100 schwannomas and neurofibromas, and transthyretin in choroid plexus papilloma. Chordomas are positive for cytokeratin, EMA, and S100.

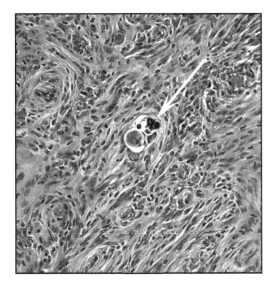

40.

C Persistent trigeminal a

Persistent trigeminal a occurs in 0.1–0.5% of cerebral angiograms. It connects the precavernous or proximal cavernous ICA to the basilar a. Note that the vessel feeds the basilar bifurcation into PCAs. It usually courses in Meckel's cave. Hypoglossal a connects cervical ICA to basilar a while proatlantal a connects ECA or cervical ICA to vertebral a. Otic (acoustic) a is rare and connects petrous ICA to basilar a.

41.

B Atlanto-occipital dislocation (AOD)

AOD is observed on CT, note the increase in the basion-dens interval on the sagittal view (normally <12 mm on X-ray) and the splaying of the joint between the occipital condyle and the lateral mass of C1, especially on the left side.

Further Reading: Martinez-Del-Campo E, Kalb S, Soriano-Baron H, et al. Computed tomography parameters for atlantooccipital dislocation in adult patients: the occipitalcondyle-C1 interval. *J Neurosurg Spine* 2016 Apr;24(4):535–545

42.

C Chordoma

Chordomas are characterized by physaliphorous (large vacuolated) cells and a mucinous background. They are common in the sacrum and clivus and are bright on T2 MRI. Surgery is the best cure. En-bloc resection should be performed whenever possible, proton beam therapy could be applied to residual tumor.

43.

B Epidermoid tumor

Epidermoid cyst, brain abscess, and infarction are bright on diffusion (restricted). Also, lymphoma, CO, prion disease, and ADEM show restricted diffusion.

44.

A A of Bernasconi and Cassinari

Presented is the typical location of the tentorial a of Bernasconi and Cassinari. It causes a blush in tentorial meningiomas. It originates from the meningohypophyseal trunk that also gives the inferior hypophyseal a and the dorsal meningeal a. Other branches of the cavernous ICA are the McConnell's capsular a and the inferior cavernous a. The superior hypophyseal a is a branch of the ophthalmic segment. The a of Percheron is a variable branch of P1 segment of the PCA and supplies both thalami.

45.

E Primary CNS lymphoma

Large B-cells with prominent nucleoli are characteristic of CNS lymphoma. Cells are CD 20+. They can be perivascular and/or intravascular. There is increased risk with AIDS. Lesions are periventricular, enhance, and show restricted diffusion.

46.

E Vein of Galen malformation

Vein of Galen malformation: well-circumscribed pineal region mass with heterogeneous signal due to blood content. Note compression of the aqueduct and hydrocephalus. They can present with heart failure in neonates or hydrocephalus later in life.

47.

D Multiple sclerosis (MS)

T2 hyperintensity on Flair MRI (frequently described as Dawson's fingers), and mild contrast enhancement in a young female are typical for MS. Symptoms are usually remittent. The blurry vision probably correlates with optic neuritis. The diagnosis can be confirmed by oligoclonal bands on lumbar puncture. Treatment includes corticosteroids, interferon beta, plasmapheresis, dimethyl fumarate (Tecfidera), ocrelizumab (Ocrevus), daclizumab (Zinbryta), and glatiramer acetate (Copaxone).

48.

A Canavan's disease

Macrocephaly is typical in Tay-Sachs disease, Canavan's disease, and Alexander's disease while microcephaly is found in Krabbe's disease (**Table 12**).

49.

C Neurofibromatosis type 2

NF2 patients develop bilateral vestibular schwannomas and meningiomas. The disease is inherited as autosomal dominant on chromosome 22.

50.

C Parkinson's disease

Lewy body (rounded pink with a halo) observed in a substantia nigra cell is typical for Parkinson's disease. Its main component is α-synuclein. Other components include ubiquitin, neurofilament, and α β crystallin.

51.

B Awake reduction with traction

The CT shows jumped facets. The patient's spine should be reduced as soon as possible using Gardner–Wells tongs or a halo ring. Reduction could be done either awake in the emergency room with serial X-rays and neurological examinations or asleep in the operating room with neurophysiological monitoring (SSEP and MEP). Prior to reduction, an MRI can be obtained to rule out acute disc herniation.

52.

B Rathke's cleft cyst

Rathke's cleft cysts have a typical MRI appearance. They are well-circumscribed intra and/or suprasellar masses, have variable signal on T1, and are usually hyperintense on T2. The pituitary gland is typically inferior to the tumor and enhances, giving it the appearance of an egg in a cup ("un œuf dans son coquetier"—French). The cysts probably arise from remnants of Rathke's pouch. Biopsy and drainage of the cyst via a transsphenoidal approach are usually sufficient to establish the diagnosis and relieve the symptoms.

Further Reading: Brassier G, Morandi X, Tayiar E, et al. Rathke's cleft cysts: surgical-MRI correlation in 16 symptomatic cases. *J Neuroradiol.* 1999;26(3):162–171

53.

A Giant thrombosed aneurysm

This well-circumscribed mass with variable signal intensity on T1 and T2 due to blood content is likely a giant thrombosed aneurysm. A vascular study (CTA, MRA, or DSA) is the next step. Stereotactic biopsy should not be offered and may cause fatal bleeding.

54.

D Incremental response to repetitive nerve stimulation

Repetitive stimulation of a motor nerve causes decremental response in myasthenia gravis (exhaustion of Ach stores) but incremental response in Lambert–Eaton myasthenic syndrome (facilitation).

55. E.

Cystic areas and Rosenthal fibers (*arrow*) are characteristic of pilocytic astrocytoma.

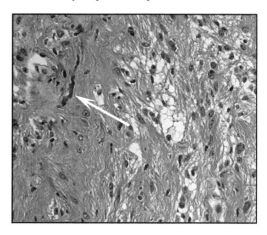

56.

E Multinucleated cells

Measles: multinucleated cells

57.

A Negri bodies

*R*abies: Neg*r*i bodies

58.

C Hirano bodies

Alzheimer's: Hirano bodies

59.

B Bunina bodies

ALS: Bunina bodies

60.

D Lewy bodies

Parkinson's: Lewy bodies

15 Test 8—Neurobiology and Neurosurgery

1.
Meissner's corpuscles have all of the following characteristics, *except*

A. Presence in the dermal papillae
B. Receptors for touch
C. Rapidly adapting
D. Small receptive field
E. Sending signals through type IV fibers

2.
The best target for DBS for essential tremors is

A. Subthalamic nucleus (STN)
B. Vim of thalamus
C. Globus pallidus internus (GPi)
D. Nucleus accumbens septi
E. Subcallosal cingulate gyrus

3.
In the dorsal horn of the spinal cord, pain sensation is transmitted by

A. Substance P and glutamate
B. Substance P and acetylcholine
C. Substance P and serotonin
D. Serotonin and glutamate
E. Norepinephrine and enkephalins

4.
Succinylcholine is a(n)

A. Ganglionic blocker
B. Depolarizing neuromuscular blocker
C. Competitive neuromuscular blocker
D. Muscarinic acetylcholine receptor inhibitor
E. Acetylcholinesterase inhibitor

5.
Peritumoral edema in meningiomas strongly correlate with high expression of

A. Epithelial membrane antigen (EMA)
B. Brain-derived neurotrophic factor (BDNF)
C. Vascular endothelial growth factor (VEGF)
D. Progesterone
E. Chondroitinase

6.
All of the following statements are true regarding Renshaw cells, *except*

A. Interneurons in the anterior horn of the spinal cord
B. Neurotransmitter serotonin
C. Efferents to alpha motor neurons
D. Afferents from alpha motor neurons
E. Inhibitory

7.
After a severe motor cycle accident, a patient has paralysis of the deltoid, infraspinatus, and biceps. The lesion most likely localizes to which part of the brachial plexus?

A. Musculocutaneous n
B. Lateral cord
C. Upper trunk
D. Middle trunk
E. Posterior cord

8.
In the previous patient, pseudomeningoceles are found on CT-myelogram. The most appropriate treatment is

A. Nerve grafting
B. Direct repair
C. Tube repair
D. Nerve transfers
E. None of the above

9.
Paccioni granulations are involved in

A. Cutaneous touch sensation
B. Hearing
C. Vision
D. CSF production
E. CSF absorption

10.
The Golgi tendon organ sends its signals through which type of fibers?

A. Ia
B. Ib
C. II
D. III
E. IV

11.

Fröhse arcade can cause entrapment of

A. Suprascapular n
B. Ulnar n
C. Anterior interosseous n (AIN)
D. Posterior interosseous n (PIN)
E. Median n

12.

Regarding core competencies, an awareness of the larger context of health care and an ability to call on resources is called

A. Practice-based learning and improvement
B. Systems-based practice
C. Interpersonal and communication skills
D. Professionalism
E. Patient care

13.

The organ of Corti responsible for hearing is located on the

A. Tympanic membrane
B. Vestibular (Reissner's) membrane
C. Basilar membrane
D. Superior olivary nucleus
E. Inferior collicullus

14.

The main mechanism of formation of secondary glioblastoma multiforme (GBM) is

A. TP53 mutation
B. LOH 10q
C. 1p19q deletion
D. PTEN mutation
E. EGFR amplification

15.

Which of the following proteins is the product of tuberous sclerosis 1 (TSC1) and is located on chromosome 9?

A. Hamartin
B. Tuberin
C. Neurofibromin
D. Tau
E. Alpha-synuclein

16.

Tetrodotoxin is a powerful blocker of

A. Cl^- channels
B. Ca^{++} channels
C. K^+ channels
D. Na^+ channels

17.

Of the medulloblastoma subgroups, which one has the best prognosis?

A. WNT
B. Sonic hedgehog (SHH)
C. Group 3
D. Group 4

18.

The depolarization part of the nerve action potential is caused by

A. K^+ influx
B. K^+ efflux
C. Ca^{++} influx
D. Na^+–K^+ pump
E. Na^+ influx

19.

Neurotransmitter release from the presynaptic terminal is caused by

A. Na^+ influx
B. Ca^{++} influx
C. K^+ influx
D. K^+ efflux
E. Closure of voltage-gated Na^+ channels

20.

The muscle stretch reflex includes all of the following components and features, *except*

A. Muscle spindle
B. Dorsal root ganglion
C. Interneuron
D. Anterior horn cell
E. It is ipsilateral and affects the same segment

21.

The rate-limiting step in dopamine synthesis uses

A. Tyrosine hydroxylase
B. L-Aromatic amino acid decarboxylase (AADC)
C. Dopamine β–hydroxylase (DBH)
D. Phenylethanolamine N-methyltransferase (PNMT)

22.

During EMG, the H-reflex

A. Is produced by supramaximal stimulation
B. Bypasses the spinal cord
C. Occurs 3–6 ms after the stimulation
D. Is the electrical equivalent of the muscle stretch reflex

23.

All of the following statements are true regarding the climbing fibers in the cerebellum, *except*

A. They arise from the inferior olivary complex
B. They are inhibitory
C. They travel through the inferior cerebellar peduncle
D. They synapse on Purkinje cell dendrites

24.

Bill's bar separates

A. The cochlear n from the inferior vestibular n
B. The facial n from the cochlear n
C. The superior and inferior vestibular nn
D. The facial n from the inferior vestibular n
E. The facial n from the superior vestibular n

25.

All of the following statements are true regarding the pelvic incidence, *except*

A. It is the angle between the perpendicular to the sacral plate at its midpoint and the line connecting the sacral plate midpoint to the axis of the femoral heads
B. It is an important parameter of sagittal balance
C. It changes as the person ages
D. It should be within <10° of lumbar lordosis
E. Its normal value is 55° ± 10°

26.

Nitric oxide (NO) has all of the following features, *except*

A. It is formed by nitric oxide synthetase (NOS)
B. It is stored in presynaptic vesicles
C. It is an unconventional neurotransmitter
D. It causes vasodilatation
E. It causes intestinal relaxation

27.

The plateau phase of the cardiac Purkinje cell action potential is caused by

A. Na^+ influx
B. Na^+ efflux
C. Ca^{++} influx
D. Ca^{++} efflux
E. K^+ influx

28.

Chorea is caused by

A. Loss of gamma-aminobutyric acid (GABA) outflow from the corpus striatum to the globus pallidus externus (GPe).
B. Loss of dopamine (DA) output from substantia nigra (SN) to the corpus striatum.
C. A lesion in the subthalamic nucleus (STN).
D. Decreased glutamate output from the cerebral cortex to the putamen.
E. Degeneration of the cerebellar dentate nucleus.

29.

The re-rupture rate after untreated aneurysmal subarachnoid hemorrhage at 2 weeks is

A. 1%
B. 5%
C. 10%
D. 20%
E. 50%

30.

At 2 years, surgical treatment of symptomatic carotid a stenosis >70% reduces the stroke risk from

A. 5% to 0%
B. 11% to 5%
C. 15% to 9%
D. 26% to 9%
E. 26% to 2%

31.

Tetraethylammonium (TEA) blocks which channels?

A. Na^+
B. Cl^-
C. Ca^{++}
D. K^+

32.

The endolymph is present in all of the following structures, *except*

A. Membranous labyrinth
B. Utricle
C. Saccule
D. Semicircular canals
E. Scala vestibuli

33.
Which of the following drugs decreases acetylcholine degradation and can be used to treat myasthenia gravis?

A.   Reserpine
B.   Phentolamine
C.   Pyridostigmine
D.   Pyridoxine
E.   Methacholine

34.
The effects of cocaine in the central nervous system are mediated by

A.   Increased dopamine (DA)
B.   Decreased dopamine
C.   Increased acetylcholine
D.   Decreased acetylcholine
E.   Decreased norepinephrine (NE)

35.
The receptors for sweating are

A.   Muscarinic acetylcholine
B.   Nicotinic acetylcholine
C.   Alpha adrenergic
D.   Beta adrenergic
E.   Serotonergic

36.
Nimodipine reduces the severity of neurological deficits from vasospasm by

A.   Direct neuromuscular blockade
B. Ca^{++} channel blockade
C.   Sympathetic ganglion blockade
D.   Alpha receptor blockade
E.   Parasympathomimetic effect

37.
The neuroleptic effects of haloperidol are caused by

A.   Blocking histamine receptors
B.   Blocking serotonin receptors
C.   Blocking α-adrenergic receptors
D.   Blocking dopamine receptors
E.   Blocking acetylcholine receptors

38.
All of the following statements are true regarding the carotid sinus reflex, *except*

A.   Caused by stimulation of baroreceptors in the carotid bulb
B.   Mediated through cranial nerve XI
C.   Relay in the brain stem
D.   Causes bradycardia
E.   Can cause death

39.
All of the following statements are true regarding Merkel's discs, *except*

A.   Present in the dermal papillae
B.   Sense vibrations
C.   Slow to adapt
D.   Have a small receptive field
E.   Signals travel through type II fibers

40.
Serotonin syndrome can be caused by any of the following drugs, *except*

A.   Duloxetine (Cymbalta)
B.   Venlafaxine (Effexor)
C.   Sumatriptan (Imitrex)
D.   Fluoxetine (Prozac)
E.   Phenytoin (Dilantin)

41.
Pedicle subtraction osteotomy (PSO) produces what degree of correction in sagittal balance?

A.   5°
B.   10°
C.   30°
D.   45°
E.   60°

42.
The most common neurological complication after lateral trans-psoas procedures for lumbar spine is

A.   Hip flexor and quadriceps weakness
B.   Hamstring weakness
C.   Foot drop
D.   Plantar flexion weakness
E.   Hip extensor weakness

43.
All of the following are true regarding Cowden's syndrome, *except*

A.   PTEN mutation
B.   Breast cancer
C.   Thyroid cancer
D.   Medulloblastoma
E.   Lhermitte–Duclos disease

44.
The normal atlantodental interval (ADI) in an adult is less than

A.   1 mm
B.   3 mm
C.   5 mm
D.   7 mm
E.   9 mm

45.
Sectioning the corpus callosum in a right-handed person can result in all of the following, *except*

A. Left-hand motor apraxia to verbal commands
B. Left auditory suppression
C. Anomia for objects in the left visual field
D. Anomia for objects in the left hand when the eyes are closed
E. Left constructional apraxia

46.
Injury to the cerebellar vermis causes

A. Truncal ataxia
B. Dysmetria
C. Hypertonia
D. Intention tremors
E. Nystagmus

47.
The efferent component of the light reflex arises from which nucleus of the oculomotor n?

A. Edinger–Westphal nucleus
B. Central nucleus
C. Medial nucleus
D. Lateral nucleus

48.
At normal intracranial pressure, autoregulation maintains a constant cerebral blood flow for changes in the mean arterial blood pressure between

A. 20 and 60 mmHg
B. 40 and 80 mmHg
C. 60 and 160 mmHg
D. 80 to 180 mmHg
E. 100–180 mmHg

49.
Myelination in the central nervous system occurs by which cells?

A. Astrocytes
B. Oligodendrocytes
C. Microglia
D. Schwann cells
E. Ependymal cells

50.
Which of the following cells are an important component of the blood–brain barrier?

A. Astrocytes
B. Oligodendrocytes
C. Microglia
D. Neurons
E. Ependymal cells

51.
A 34-year-old male with history of diabetes mellitus, alcohol abuse, and hemochromatosis presents with right eye swelling, proptosis, and ophthalmoplegia together with diabetic ketoacidosis. This progressed to blindness within 3 days. He then developed headache, nuchal rigidity, and confusion. The patient died within 3 weeks despite maximum surgical and medical management. The MRI images are shown below. The most likely diagnosis is

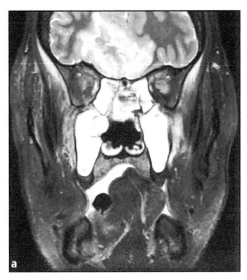

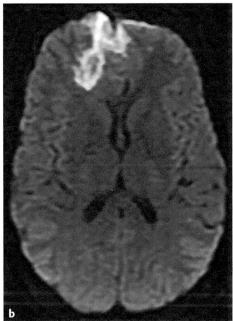

A. Staphylococcal brain abscess
B. Meningococcal meningitis
C. Herpes encephalitis
D. Mucormycosis
E. Gliomatosis cerebri

52.

A 68-year-old male presents 6 hours after dense left hemiparesis with the following CT head. The patient is awake and follows commands with the right side. The most important next step in this patient management that will affect his functional recovery is

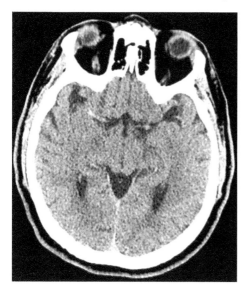

A. Right decompressive hemicraniectomy
B. Endovascular coiling
C. Intra-arterial thrombolysis
D. Intravenous tPA
E. Intravenous heparin

53.

In the following endoscopic view of the lateral ventricle, the fornix is represented by number

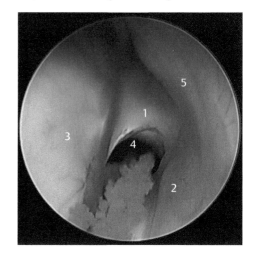

A. 1
B. 2
C. 3
D. 4
E. 5

54.

The nerve supply to the skin of the dorsum of the first web space of the foot is

A. Sural n
B. Saphenous n
C. Medial plantar n
D. Superficial peroneal n
E. Deep peroneal n

55.

The best medical treatment of Paget's disease of the spine includes

A. Parathyroid hormone (PTH)
B. Bisphosphonates
C. Calcium supplements
D. Methotrexate
E. Azathioprine

56.

Which of the following nuclei correspond with Lateral amygdala to cerebral cortex?

A. Glycine
B. GABA
C. Acetylcholine
D. Dopamine
E. 5-HT (serotonin)

57.

Which of the following nuclei correspond with Dorsal raphe nucleus?

A. Glycine
B. GABA
C. Acetylcholine
D. Dopamine
E. 5-HT (serotonin)

58.

Which of the following nuclei correspond with Globus pallidus externus to subthalamic nucleus?

A. Glycine
B. GABA
C. Acetylcholine
D. Dopamine
E. 5-HT (serotonin)

59.

Which of the following nuclei correspond with Renshaw cells?

A. Glycine
B. GABA
C. Acetylcholine
D. Dopamine
E. 5-HT (serotonin)

60.

Which of the following nuclei correspond with Substantia nigra, pars compacta?

A. Glycine
B. GABA
C. Acetylcholine
D. Dopamine
E. 5-HT (serotonin)

16 Answer Key 8

1.

E Sending signals through type IV fibers

Meissner's corpuscles transmit touch and vibration and send signals through type II fibers. Type IV fibers are mainly for pain and temperature (**Table 2**).

2.

B Ventral intermediate nucleus of thalamus (Vim)

DBS targets for: Parkinsonism → STN, essential tremors → Vim, dystonia → GPi, nucleus accumbens septi → obsessive-compulsive disorder (OCD), subcallosal cingulate gyrus → depression.

3.

A Substance P and glutamate

The neurotransmitters for pain in the dorsal horn are substance P (chronic pain, burning, slow) and glutamate (acute pain, sharp, fast). Enkephalins are secreted by interneurons and inhibit pain (**Fig. 15**).

4.

B Depolarizing neuromuscular blocker

Succinylcholine is a paralytic used with general anesthesia, works by persistent depolarization of the neuromuscular junction. Pentolinium is a ganglionic (nicotinic acetylcholine receptor) blocker used to treat hypertension. Curare derivatives are competitive neuromuscular blockers. Atropine is a muscarinic acetylcholine receptor inhibitor. Acetylcholinesterase inhibitors (anticholinesterases), like neostigmine, are used to treat myasthenia gravis (**Fig. 25**).

5.

C Vascular endothelial growth factor (VEGF)

Meningiomas with severe peritumoral edema express high levels of vascular endothelial growth factor (VEGF) and matrix metalloproteinases (MMPs).

Further Reading: Paek SH, Kim CY, Kim YY, et al. Correlation of clinical and biological parameters with peritumoral edema in meningioma. *J Neurooncol*. 2002 Dec;60(3):235–245

6.

B Neurotransmitter serotonin

Renshaw cells are interneurons in the Rexed laminae VII and VIII in the spinal cord. They provide recurrent inhibition to the α-motor neuron. They release glycine, which opens chloride channels. Strychnine is a glycine antagonist; it causes rigidity while tetanus prevents the release of glycine (**Figs. 26 and 27**).

7.

C Upper trunk

The upper trunk (C5, C6) of the brachial plexus divides into suprascapular n (**S**) (supraspinatus and infraspinatus), posterior division (**P**) (axillary n, deltoid), and anterior division (**A**) (musculocutaneous n, biceps), hence the mnemonic **SPA** (**Fig. 16**).

Further Reading: Hanna A. The SPA arrangement of the branches of the upper trunk of the brachial plexus: a correction of a longstanding misconception and a new diagram of the brachial plexus. *J Neurosurg* 2016 Aug;125(2):350–354

8.

D Nerve transfers

Pseudomeningoceles most likely signify brachial plexus avulsion. Since these are preganglionic lesions, the best treatment involves nerve transfers. These include ulnar n fascicle to musculocutaneous n (Oberlin transfer), intercostal nn to musculocutaneous n, triceps branch (of radial n) to axillary n, and spinal XI to suprascapular n.

9.

E CSF absorption

Paccioni granulations are arachnoid villi that filter the cerebrospinal fluid from the subarachnoid space to the venous sinuses.

10.

B Ib

Golgi tendon organ is stimulated by active muscle contraction or strong passive stretch. It sends signals through Ib (Aα) fibers at 120 m/s. This results in stimulation of Renshaw cells which in turn inhibit α-motor neurons by releasing glycine which opens chloride channels (**Table 1, Fig. 28**).

11.

D Posterior interosseous n (PIN)

The arcade of Fröhse is the edge of the supinator and can compress the PIN. The suprascapular n can be compressed by the suprascapular ligament, the ulnar n by the Osborne band, the arcade of Struthers, or in the Guyon's canal, the AIN by the pronator teres or the flexor digitorum superficialis (sublime) arch, and the *m*edian n by the liga*m*ent of Struthers, pronator teres, sublime arch, or transverse carpal ligament.

12.

B Systems-based practice

The 6 Accreditation Council for Graduate Medical Education (ACGME) core competencies are:

Patient care	Compassionate, appropriate, and effective care for the treatment of health problems and the promotion of health.
Medical knowledge	Knowledge about established and evolving biomedical, clinical, and cognate (e.g., epidemiological and social-behavioral) sciences and the application of this knowledge to patient care.
Practice-based learning and improvement	Investigation and evaluation of patient care practices, appraisal and assimilation of scientific evidence, and improvements in patient care.
Interpersonal and communication skills	Effective information exchange and teaming with patients, families, and professional associates.
Professionalism	A commitment to carrying out professional responsibilities, adherence to ethical principles, and sensitivity to a diverse patient population.
Systems-based practice	An awareness of and responsiveness to the larger context and system of healthcare and the ability to effectively call on system resources to provide care that is of optimal value.

13.

C Basilar membrane

The organ of Corti is composed of hair cells responsible for hearing. These are located on the basilar membrane that separates scala tympani from scala media and their cilia project into the tectorial membrane. Activation of the hair cells stimulates the cochlear nerve endings. The vestibular (Reissner's) membrane separates scala media from scala vestibuli.

14.

A TP53 mutation

TP53 mutations are early and frequent genetic alterations in the pathway leading to secondary glioblastomas (65%) while PTEN mutation (25%) and EGFR amplification (36%) occur in primary GBM. LOH 10q is common in both (**Table 6**). Co-deletion of 1p19q occurs in oligodendrogliomas.

Further Reading: Ohgaki H, Kleihues P. Genetic pathways to primary and secondary glioblastoma. *Am J Pathol.* 2007 May;170(5):1445–1453

Ohgaki H, Kleihues P. Population-based studies on incidence, survival rates, and genetic alterations in astrocytic and oligodendroglial gliomas. *J Neuropathol Exp Neurol.* 2005 Jun;64(6):479–489

15.

A Hamartin

Hamartin is the byproduct of TSC1 (chromosome 9) and tuberin is from TSC2 (chromosome 16) (**Table 11**). Neurofibromin is associated with neurofibromatosis. Tau protein is associated with Alzheimer's disease causing neurofibrillary tangles. Alpha-synuclein is found in Lewy bodies seen in Parkinson's disease.

Further Reading: Plank TL, Yeung RS, Henske EP. Hamartin, the product of the tuberous sclerosis 1 (TSC1) gene, interacts with tuberin and appears to be localized to cytoplasmic vesicles. *Cancer Res.* 1998 Nov 1;58(21):4766–4770

16.

D Na+ channels

Tetrodotoxin (TTX), a powerful poison in the Spheroides rubripes (puffer fish), selectively blocks voltage-dependent sodium channels. It prevents depolarization and propagation of nerve action potential. Saxitoxin found in shellfish has a similar effect and causes paralytic shellfish poisoning (**Fig. 27**).

17.

A WNT

In the medulloblastoma subtypes, WNT has the best prognosis with a 5-year overall survival of 95% in children and 100% in adults. Group 3 has the worst prognosis.

Further Reading: Bourdeaut F, Pouponnot C, Ayrault O. Les médulloblastomes et leurs cellules d'origine (Subtypes of medulloblastomas: distinct cellular origins). *Med Sci.* (Paris) 2012 Oct;28(10):805–809

Kool M, Korshunov A, Remke M, et al. Molecular subgroups of medulloblastoma: an international meta-analysis of transcriptome, genetic aberrations, and clinical data of WNT, SHH, Group 3, and Group 4 medulloblastomas. *Acta Neuropathol.* 2012 Apr;123(4):473–484

18.

E Na+ influx

Rush of Na+ inside the nerve causes its depolarization. Repolarization is caused by K+ efflux while the Na+ channels are closed. The Na+-K+ pump is an ATP-dependent mechanism to maintain a high concentration of Na+ outside the cell and K+ inside the cell at the resting state. The axon hillock has the largest concentration of Na+ channels and is the most excitable part of the neuron (**Fig. 27**).

19.

B Ca++ influx

Once the action potential reaches the axon terminal, it activates Ca++ channels. Ca++ influx causes synaptic vesicles to fuse with the presynaptic membrane through SNARE complex and release neurotransmitters by exocytosis. Neurotransmitters are inactivated by reuptake or degradation. In Lambert–Eaton myasthenic syndrome (LEMS), antibodies inhibit presynaptic voltage-gated calcium channels (VGCC) while botulinum toxin inhibits SNARE (**Fig. 26**).

20.

C Interneuron

The muscle stretch reflex is monosynaptic, no interneurons are involved (**Fig. 28**).

21.

A Tyrosine hydroxylase

Tyrosine hydroxylase mediates the transformation of tyrosine to L-dihydroxyphenylalanine (L-DOPA). It is the rate-limiting step in catecholamine synthesis because TH saturates with tyrosine. L-Aromatic amino acid decarboxylase transforms L-DOPA to dopamine (DA). Dopamine β–hydroxylase transforms DA to norepinephrine (NE). Phenylethanolamine N-methyltransferase transforms NE to epinephrine.

22.

D Is the electrical equivalent of the muscle stretch reflex

The H-reflex (Hoffmann's reflex) on EMG is the electrical equivalent of the muscle stretch reflex. It occurs 28–35 ms after submaximal stimulation, goes through the spinal cord, and afferents travel through Ia fibers. The M-wave is a direct motor response at 3–6 ms that bypasses the spinal cord. Supramaximal stimulation is used to generate an F-response through antidromic activation of α- motor neurons (**Fig. 27**).

Further Reading: Chen YS, Zhou S. Soleus H-reflex and its relation to static postural control. *Gait Posture* 2011 Feb;33(2):169–178

Palmieri RM, Ingersoll CD, Hoffman MA. The Hoffmann reflex: methodologic considerations and applications for use in sports medicine and athletic training research. *J Athl Train.* 2004 Jul;39(3):268–277

23.

B They are inhibitory.

The climbing fibers are excitatory, secrete glutamate, arise from the contralateral inferior olivary complex, travel through the inferior cerebellar peduncle, and synapse on Purkinje cell dendrites and to a lesser extent granule cell parallel fibers, basket and stellate cells. In the cerebellum, climbing fibers, mossy fibers, and granule cells are excitatory (**Fig. 11**).

24.

E The facial n from the superior vestibular n

Bill's bar separates facial n from superior vestibular n (**Fig. 14**).

25.

C It changes as the person ages.

The pelvic incidence is essentially constant.

Further Reading: Rose PS, Bridwell KH, Lenke LG, et al. Role of pelvic incidence, thoracic kyphosis, and patient factors on sagittal plane correction following pedicle subtraction osteotomy. *Spine* 2009 Apr 15;34(8):785–791

Le Huec JC, Aunoble S, Philippe L, Nicolas P. Pelvic parameters: origin and significance. *Eur Spine J.* 2011 Sep;20(Suppl 5):564–571

Legaye J, Duval-Beaupère G, Hecquet J, Marty C. Pelvic incidence: a fundamental pelvic parameter for three-dimensional regulation of spinal sagittal curves. *Eur Spine J.* 1998;7(2):99–103

26.

B It is stored in presynaptic vesicles.

Nitric oxide is an unconventional transmitter since it is not stored in cells, is not released by exocytosis, does not act on specific receptors, and lacks a specific inactivation process.

27.

C Ca^{++} influx

The plateau phase in the cardiac muscle action potential is caused by a slow Ca^{++} influx along with a K^+ efflux. Depolarization is caused by Na^+ influx, while repolarization is caused by K^+ efflux (**Fig. 27**).

28.

A Loss of gamma-aminobutyric acid (GABA) outflow from the corpus striatum to the globus pallidus externus (GPe).

Chorea is caused by loss of gamma-aminobutyric acid (GABA) outflow from the striatum to the globus pallidus externus (GPe). Parkinson's disease is caused by loss of dopamine (DA) output from substantia nigra (SN) to the striatum. Hemiballismus is caused by an injury in the contralateral STN (**Fig. 7**).

29.

D 20%

The re-rupture rate after untreated aneurysmal subarachnoid hemorrhage is 20% at 2 weeks (highest within the first 24 hours) and 50% at 6 months.

30.

D 26% to 9%

Based on NASCET (North American Symptomatic Carotid Endarterectomy Trial), surgical treatment of symptomatic carotid a stenosis ≥70% resulted in reducing the stroke risk from 26% to 9% at 2 years. Based on ACAS (Asymptomatic Carotid Atherosclerosis Study), carotid endarterectomy resulted in reduced stroke risk from 11% to 5% over 5 years for stenosis ≥60%.

Further Reading: North American Symptomatic Carotid Endarterectomy Trial Collaborators. Beneficial effect of carotid endarterectomy in symptomatic patients with high-grade carotid stenosis. *N Engl J Med.* 1991;325:445–453

Executive Committee for the Asymptomatic Carotid Atherosclerosis Study. Endarterectomy for asymptomatic carotid artery stenosis. *JAMA* 1995;273(18): 1421–1428

31.

D K^+

Tetraethylammonium is a ganglion blocker. It inhibits nicotinic acetylcholine receptors and K^+ channels in autonomic ganglia. It can cause vasodilatation (**Fig. 25**).

32.

E Scala vestibuli

The endolymph fills up the membranous labyrinth, including scala media. Its composition is similar to the intracellular fluid and it plays a role in both the auditory and the vestibular systems. The perilymph is between the membranous labyrinth and the bony labyrinth. It fills up the scala vestibuli and the scala tympani.

33.

C Pyridostigmine

Pyridostigmine is a reversible anticholinesterase used for myasthenia gravis. **Res**erpine is an antihypertensive drug that blocks the **s**ynthe**s**is and **s**torage of no**r**epineph**r**ine and **ser**otonin. Phentolamine is also an antihypertensive through competitive non-selective α-adrenergic antagonism (**Fig. 25**). Methacholine is a parasympathomimetic which causes bronchospasm, and is used to test for asthma. Pyridoxine is vitamin B6.

34.

A Increased dopamine (DA)

Cocaine blocks the uptake and transport of dopamine (DA), norepinephrine (NE), and serotonin

(5-HT). It produces its "high" effects by causing excessive levels of dopamine in the brain. It is also used as a local anesthetic by blocking Na⁺ channels and as a vasoconstrictor.

35.

A   Muscarinic acetylcholine

Sweating, despite being a sympathetic function, is mediated by muscarinic acetylcholine receptors (**Fig. 25**).

36.

B   Ca⁺⁺ channel blockade

Nimodipine is a L-type voltage-gated Ca⁺⁺ channel blocker, thus inhibiting vascular smooth muscle contraction. It should be given prophylactically after aneurysmal subarachnoid hemorrhage to help prevent serious consequences of cerebral vasospasm. Dose is 60 mg orally every 4 hours for 3 weeks.

Further Reading: Allen GS, Ahn HS, Preziosi TJ. Cerebral arterial spasm—a controlled trial of nimodipine in patients with subarachnoid hemorrhage. *N Engl J Med.* 1983 Mar 17;308(11):619–624

37.

D   Blocking dopamine receptors

Haloperidol is a powerful neuroleptic (antipsychotic), used to treat schizophrenia, by blocking dopamine receptors in the limbic system. Side effects are caused by blocking histaminergic, serotonergic, and α-adrenergic receptors.

38.

B   Mediated through cranial nerve XI

Carotid sinus reflex afferents: IX (Hering's n), efferents X (**Fig. 14**).

Further Reading: Krediet CT, Parry SW, Jardine DL, Benditt DG, Brignole M, Wieling W. The history of diagnosing carotid sinus hypersensitivity: why are the current criteria too sensitive? *Europace* 2011 Jan;13(1):4–22

39.

B.   Sense vibrations

Merkel's discs transmit touch and pressure sensations (**Table 2**).

40.

E   Phenytoin (Dilantin

Serotonin syndrome is a serious interaction when two or more serotonergic drugs are used. Symptoms include agitation, dilated pupils, tachycardia, diarrhea, sweating, fever, seizures, and death. Causes include Prozac (fluoxetine) (a selective serotonin reuptake inhibitor), Cymbalta and Effexor (5-HT and NE reuptake inhibitors), amitriptyline (a tricyclic antidepressant), monoamine oxidase inhibitors, and anti-migraine medications (Imitrex). Phenytoin is an anti-epileptic drug that does not increase serotonin levels, it works by Na⁺ channel blockade.

41.

C   30°

PSO creates a wedge in the vertebral body and achieves 30°–35° of sagittal balance correction. It is usually performed in the mid-lumbar spine (L3 or L2). Ponte osteotomy creates a wedge in the lamina and facets and achieves 10°–15° correction per level. Smith–Peterson osteotomy (SPO) in addition creates a distraction opening of the anterior longitudinal ligament, thus increasing the risk of vascular injuries. For optimal deformity correction, pelvic incidence–lumbar lordosis should be <10°.

Further Reading: Kim KT, Park KJ, Lee JH. Osteotomy of the spine to correct the spinal deformity. *Asian Spine J.* 2009 Dec;3(2):113–123

Bridwell KH. Decision making regarding Smith–Petersen vs. pedicle subtraction osteotomy vs. vertebral column resection for spinal deformity. *Spine* 2006 Sep 1;31(19 Suppl):S171–178

42.

A   Hip flexor and quadriceps weakness

The incidence of hip flexor and quadriceps weakness after lateral trans-psoas procedures (DLIF: direct lateral interbody fusion, or XLIF: extreme lateral interbody fusion) is 25%. This is due to damage to the lumbar plexus and/or the psoas muscle.

43.

D   Medulloblastoma

Cowden's syndrome is an autosomal dominant multiple hamartoma syndrome with mutation of PTEN, a tumor-suppressor gene on chromosome 10q. It affects 1 in 200,000 people. It can cause Lhermitte–Duclos disease, breast, thyroid, and uterine cancer (**Table 11**).

44.

B   3 mm

The normal ADI is less than 3 mm in adults, 5 mm in children. However, recent CT data suggest that the normal interval in most normal adults is less than 2 mm.

45.

E Left constructional apraxia

One of the main risks of corpus callosotomy is disconnection syndrome. Constructional apraxia is inability to perform tasks requiring spatial processing (e.g., copying geometric forms). This is processed in the right hemisphere. Therefore, in disconnection syndrome, the left hand is intact but the right hand is affected. A, C and D are left hemispheric functions, they are normal on the right side of the body and lost on the left side. If different words are presented to each ear simultaneously (dichotically), the left ear signal is suppressed by the stronger contralateral signal.

46.

A Truncal ataxia

Injury to the vermis causes truncal ataxia and hypotonia. Dysmetria and intention tremors are caused by injury to the neocerebellum (lateral zone and dentate nucleus). Nystagmus is caused by injury to the flocculonodular lobe.

Further Reading: Bodranghien F, Bastian A, Casali C, et al. Consensus paper: revisiting the symptoms and signs of cerebellar syndrome. *Cerebellum* 2016 Jun;15(3):369–391

47.

A Edinger–Westphal nucleus

Parasympathetic preganglionic efferents of the light reflex arise from the Edinger–Westphal nucleus of the oculomotor n (III). They travel bilaterally through the inferior division of III to relay in the ciliary ganglion and supply the constrictor pupillae muscle causing the direct (ipsilateral) and consensual (contralateral) light reflex. The central nucleus supplies the levator palpebrae superioris bilaterally, the medial nucleus the contralateral superior rectus, and the lateral nucleus the ipsilateral inferior oblique, medial rectus, and inferior rectus (**Fig. 14**).

48.

C 60 and 160 mmHg

Cerebral autoregulation maintains a constant cerebral blood flow despite fluctuations in mean arterial blood pressure (MAP): If the systemic blood pressure drops, the brain vessels dilate to accommodate more blood; if the blood pressure is high the cerebral blood vessels constrict. Autoregulation fails at extremes of MAP. The exact number varies according to the source. Some say that the range of autoregulation is MAP 60–160 mmHg, some MAP 50–150 mmHg, and others CPP 60–160 mmHg. Note that CPP = MAP – ICP and MAP = DBP + 1/3 (SBP – DBP); where CPP, cerebral perfusion pressure; ICP, intracranial pressure; DBP, diastolic blood pressure; SBP, systolic blood pressure.

49.

B Oligodendrocytes

Oligodendrocytes myelinate the CNS, while Schwann cells myelinate the peripheral nervous system. The transition zone between central myelin and peripheral myelin is called the Obersteiner–Redlich zone. This was once thought to be where vestibular nerve schwannomas originate. However, most tumors actually originate lateral to this zone.

50.

A Astrocytes

The main components of the blood–brain barrier (BBB) are vascular endothelial cells with their tight junctions and basement membranes as well as astrocytic foot processes. Most circumventricular organs are deficient in blood–brain barrier: **p**ineal gland, median eminence and **p**osterior pituitary, area **p**ostrema (paired), organum vasculosum of the lamina terminalis, and subforniceal organ. The only circumventricular organ with intact BBB is the subcommissural organ (**Fig. 24B**).

51.

D Mucormycosis

Aggressive rhinocerebral mucormycosis (zygomycosis or phycomycosis) occurs in patients with poorly controlled diabetes mellitus. **a.** Coronal T2 fat suppressed MRI shows involvement of bilateral nasal sinuses and frontal lobes. **b.** Axial cut shows diffusion restriction. Treatment includes surgical debridement and antifungals. Prognosis is poor. Herpes encephalitis preferentially affects medial temporal lobes. *Staphylococcus aureus* is common after neurosurgical procedures or trauma. Meningococcal meningitis is common in school age (children and young adults), especially in poor crowded areas like sub-Saharan Africa. The incidence is less after widespread vaccination.

52.

C   Intra-arterial thrombolysis

Hyperdense right MCA sign seen on the CT is a sign of ischemic stroke. The patient's symptoms are >4.5 hours which is out of the window for IV tPA (0.9 mg/kg [maximum 90 mg], 10% of dose as IV bolus over 1 minute). He is still a candidate for intra-arterial revascularization (tPA or mechanical thrombectomy). Decompressive hemicraniectomy is not indicated since the patient is wide awake with no midline shift.

Further Reading: Berkhemer OA, Fransen PS, Beumer D, et al. A randomized trial of intraarterial treatment for acute ischemic stroke. *N Engl J Med.* 2015;372(1):11–20

Campbell BC, Mitchell PJ, Kleinig TJ, et al. Endovascular therapy for ischemic stroke with perfusion-imaging selection. *N Engl J Med.* 2015;372(11):1009–1018

Goyal M, Demchuk AM, Menon BK, et al. Randomized assessment of rapid endovascular treatment of ischemic stroke. *N Engl J Med.* 2015;372(11):1019–1030

53.

A   1

Endoscopic view of the right lateral ventricle. 1, fornix: forms the superior and anterior boundary of the foramen of Monro (4). The choroid plexus is observed between the septum pellucidum (3) and thalamus (2); 5, head of caudate.

54.

E   Deep peroneal n

The majority of the dorsum of the foot is supplied by the superficial peroneal n, except for the first web space, which is supplied by the deep peroneal n. The sural n supplies the lateral aspect of the foot toward the little toe. The saphenous n (femoral n branch) supplies the area of the medial malleolus. The medial and lateral plantar nn (tibial n branches) supply the sole of the foot.

55.

B   Bisphosphonates

Bisphosphonates like pamidronate as well as calcitonin (salmon-derived) are used to treat severe Paget's disease. Patients usually have hypercalcemia and hypercalciuria and are prone to kidney stones. Lab work also shows increased serum alkaline phosphatase and urine hydroxyproline. PTH increases serum calcium and is contraindicated.

56.

C   Acetylcholine

Acetylcholine is the main output from the lateral amygdala to the cerebral cortex. This is lost in Alzheimer's disease. Aricept (donepezil) is an acetylcholinesterase inhibitor that can improve symptoms of dementia (**Fig. 7**).

57.

E   5-HT (serotonin)

Output from the dorsal raphe nucleus (DRN) to substantia nigra includes 5-HT and cholecystokinine and to the corpus striatum includes 5-HT and enkephalins (**Fig. 7**). DRN is involved in non-REM sleep (**Fig. 31**).

58.

B   GABA

Output from GPe to STN is GABA, from GPe to GPi is GABA and substance P, and from GPi to thalamus GABA (**Fig. 7**).

59.

A   Glycine

Renshaw cells are inhibitory to motor neurons in the spinal cord through the neurotransmitter glycine, which increases chloride influx. Tetanus inhibits the release of glycine, while strychnine inhibits glycine receptors, both leading to contractures (**Figs. 26** and **27**).

60.

D   Dopamine

Substantia nigra pars compacta exerts its effect on corpus striatum through dopamine (DA1 is excitatory and DA2 is inhibitory). Tyrosine hydroxylase catalyzes the rate-limiting step in catecholamine synthesis. SN degeneration causes Parkinson's disease (**Fig. 7**). Treatment includes L-dopa.

17 Test 9—Comprehensive

1.

A 52-year-old female, non-smoker, presents with double vision, bitemporal hemianopsia, and the following imaging findings. What is the most likely diagnosis?

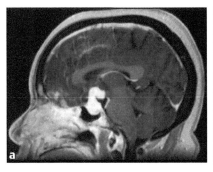 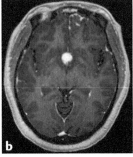 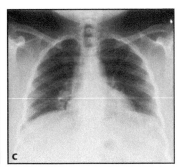

A. Lymphocytic hypophysitis
B. Metastatic lung cancer
C. Sarcoidosis
D. Pituitary macroadenoma
E. Pituitary carcinoma

2.

The substantia gelatinosa of Rolando is continuous with which trigeminal nucleus?

A. Spinal nucleus
B. Main sensory nucleus
C. Motor nucleus
D. Mesencephalic nucleus
E. None of the above

3.

The following is true about Merkel's discs, *except*

A. Present in dermal papillae of hairy and non-hairy skin
B. Transmit touch and pressure sensation
C. Slowly adapting receptors
D. Small receptive field
E. Signals travel through type III and IV fibers

4.

Arsenic poisoning is associated with all of the following, *except*

A. Mees' white lines in the nails
B. Basophilic stippling of RBCs
C. Peripheral neuropathy
D. Encephalopathy
E. Hyperkeratosis of palms and soles

5.
A 70-year-old diabetic male, with a history of myelodysplastic syndrome for which he underwent chemotherapy, presents with headaches and mental status changes. What diagnosis is supported by the following MRI findings (a, T1 with contrast; b, diffusion; and c, ADC)?

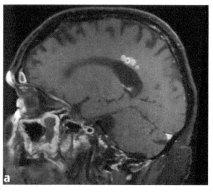 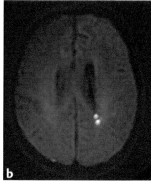 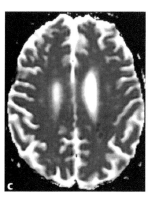

A.   Multifocal glioblastoma (GBM)
B.   Brain metastases
C.   Tumefactive multiple sclerosis (MS)
D.   Brain abscesses
E.   Epidermoid cysts

6.
Orbitofrontal syndrome is characterized by all of the following, *except*

A.   Bilateral lesions of the orbitofrontal cortex
B.   Severe cognitive decline
C.   Hypersexuality
D.   Hyperphagia
E.   Urinary behavioral disorder

7.
Following anterior cervical discectomy and fusion (ACDF) with iliac crest bone graft, a patient complains of anterolateral thigh pain; this is most likely associated with injury to the

A.   Lateral femoral cutaneous n
B.   Ilioinguinal n
C.   Genitofemoral n
D.   Intermediate cutaneous n of the thigh
E.   Posterior cutaneous n of the thigh

8.
All of the following is true about propofol (diprivan), *except*

A.   Can cause severe respiratory depression
B.   Hypertension is a known side effect
C.   Rapid acting sedative
D.   Lipid-soluble
E.   No analgesic effects

9.
The presence of macrocephaly, mental retardation, seizures, and Rosenthal fibers are characteristics of which metabolic disorder?

A.   Alexander's disease
B.   Krabbe's disease
C.   Metachromatic leukodystrophy
D.   Adrenoleukodystrophy
E.   Pilocytic astrocytoma

10.
Which of the following is true about the nucleus of tractus solitarius?

A.   Fibers travel through cranial nerves IX, X, and XI
B.   Provides general visceral efferents
C.   Provides special visceral afferents
D.   Provides general somatic efferents
E.   Provides general somatic afferents

11.

A 48-year-old female on oral contraceptive pills presents with severe headache, nausea, and vomiting. CT head axial without (**a**) and coronal with contrast (**b**) are depicted below. The most important next step in this patient's management is

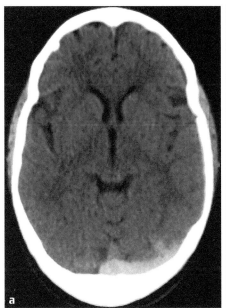 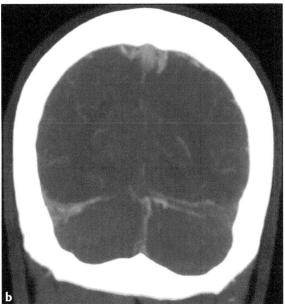

A. Aspirin (Acetylsalicylic acid)
B. Prophylactic dose of heparin subcutaneously
C. IV heparin
D. Nimodipine
E. Craniotomy

12.

After a lymph node biopsy of the neck, a patient experiences inability to raise the arm above the head and pain. His wife noticed a winged scapula. What is the most likely injured nerve?

A. Long thoracic n
B. Spinal accessory n
C. Axillary n
D. Suprascapular n
E. Upper trunk of the brachial plexus

13.

Regarding Tolosa–Hunt syndrome, the following is the *least* likely to occur

A. Periorbital headache
B. Loss of sensation over the forehead
C. Blindness
D. Third nerve palsy
E. Fourth nerve palsy

14.

A 62-year-old male presents with back pain. T2 (**a**)
and T1-contrasted (**b**) MR images reveal

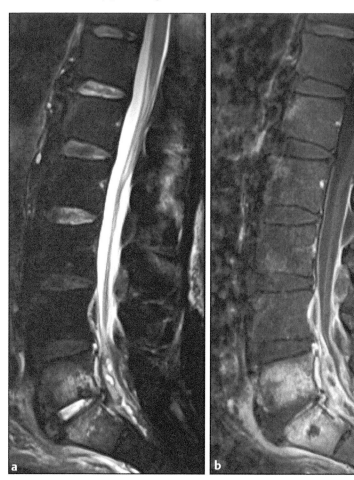

A.   Metastatic spine disease
B.   Degenerative disc disease
C.   Myxopapillary ependymoma
D.   Discitis with epidural abscess
E.   Cystic schwannoma

15.

To diagnose Creutzfeldt–Jakob disease (CJD), the
presence of which of the following in CSF is helpful?

A.   14-3-3 protein
B.   ACE (angiotensin-converting enzyme)
C.   Oligoclonal bands
D.   Placental alkaline phosphatase (PLAP)
E.   Alpha-fetoprotein (AFP)

16.

Which of the following nuclei are involved in parasympathetic control?

A. Anterior hypothalamus
B. Posterior hypothalamus
C. Lateral hypothalamus
D. Supraoptic nuclei
E. Paraventricular nuclei

17.

Stiff-man syndrome is associated with

A. Phytanic acid oxidase deficiency
B. Decreased dystrophin
C. Myophosphorylase deficiency
D. Anti-Hu antibodies
E. Anti-GAD (glutamic acid decarboxylase) antibodies

18.

A 22-year-old male presents with left-sided proptosis. The most likely diagnosis is

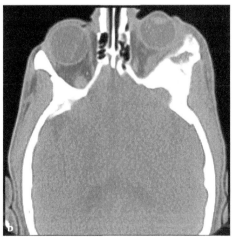

A. Metastasis
B. Meningioma
C. Eosinophilic granuloma
D. Fibrous dysplasia
E. Paget's disease

19.

All of the following is true about cerebral salt wasting syndrome (CSWS), *except*

A. Hyponatremia
B. Hypervolemia
C. Increased serum atrial natriuretic peptide (ANP)
D. Increased fractional excretion of sodium (FeNa)
E. Observed in traumatic brain injury and subarachnoid hemorrhage

20.

The following findings in a clival lesion are characteristic of

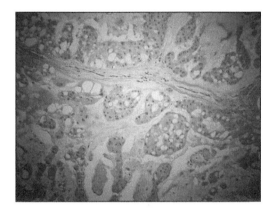

A. Chondrosarcoma
B. Chordoma
C. Metastatic lung cancer
D. Meningioma
E. Osteosarcoma

21.

Sacral sparing in the setting of a spinal cord injury

A. Is a good prognostic sign
B. Should be retested after return of the bulbocavernosus reflex
C. Is evidenced by plantar flexion of the big toe
D. Is positive if there is preserved anal sphincter function
E. All of the above

22.

The resting membrane potential is maintained by the

A. Sodium-potassium pump
B. Rapid influx of sodium
C. Calcium influx
D. Potassium efflux

23.
The following specimen was removed from the temporal lobe of a child with seizures. What is the diagnosis?

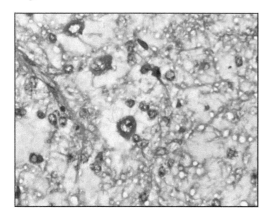

A. Ganglioglioma
B. DNET (dysembryoplastic neuroepithelial tumor)
C. Oligodendroglioma
D. Central neurocytoma
E. PNET (primitive neuroectodermal tumor)

24.
The highest Cho:NAA ratio (choline:N-acetylaspartate) on MR spectroscopy is found in

A. Normal brain
B. Ependymoma
C. Benign astrocytoma
D. Medulloblastoma
E. Radiation necrosis

25.
Dementia, diarrhea, and dermatitis may occur in which vitamin deficiency?

A. B1 (Thiamine)
B. B3 (Niacin)
C. B6 (Pyridoxine)
D. B12 (Cobalamin)
E. A

26.
Which of the following structures pass through the foramen ovale?

A. Trochlear n (IV)
B. Ophthalmic division of trigeminal n (V_1)
C. Maxillary division of trigeminal n (V_2)
D. Mandibular division of trigeminal n (V_3)
E. Middle meningeal a

27.
Wave IV of the brain auditory evoked responses (BAER) originates from

A. Cochlear nuclei
B. Superior olivary nucleus
C. Lateral lemniscus
D. Medial geniculate body
E. Auditory radiation

28.
Which brain tumor is commonly encountered in Li–Fraumeni syndrome?

A. Astrocytic glioma
B. Medulloblastoma
C. Ependymoma
D. Hemangioblastoma
E. Pituitary adenoma

29.
All of the following is true about Huntington's disease, *except*

A. CAG trinucleotide repeats
B. Autosomal recessive
C. Age 30–50 years at presentation
D. Choreiform movements and dementia
E. Striatal atrophy causing box car ventricles

30.
Suprascapular n entrapment is associated with loss of which shoulder movement?

A. Flexion
B. Extension
C. Protraction
D. Internal rotation
E. External rotation

31.
All of the following is true about abrupt intrathecal baclofen withdrawal, *except*

A. A life-threatening condition
B. Flaccidity
C. Seizures
D. Fever
E. Altered level of consciousness

32.

The lateral spinothalamic tract has all of the following features, *except*

A. It conveys pain and temperature sensation
B. It arises from the contralateral side of the body
C. Fibers originate in Rexed layers I, IV, and V
D. It is somatotopically organized with the leg medial
E. Efferents relay in the VPL (ventral posterolateral) nucleus of thalamus

33.

The first web space on the dorsum of the foot is supplied by

A. Saphenous n
B. Superficial peroneal n
C. Deep peroneal n
D. Sural n
E. Tibial n

34.

Huntington's disease is characterized by deficiency of the enzyme

A. Choline acetyltransferase
B. Acetylcholine esterase
C. Arylsulfatase B
D. Sphingomyelinase
E. Iduronate-2-sulfatase

35.

The following specimen is from an intraventricular tumor. What is the diagnosis?

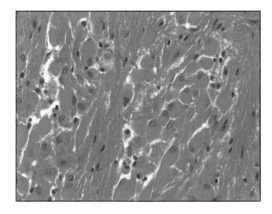

A. Ependymoma
B. Plasmacytoma
C. Meningioma
D. Medulloblastoma
E. SEGA (subependymal giant cell astrocytoma)

36.

An 18-year-old athletic female presents with low back pain. The most likely cause is

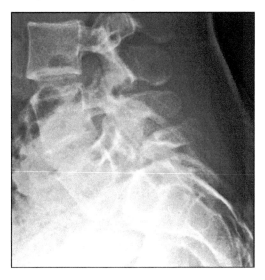

A. Spondylolysis
B. Discitis
C. Spondyloptosis
D. Spondylosis
E. Ankylosing spondylitis

37.

All of the following is true about internuclear ophthalmoplegia (INO), *except*

A. It is caused by a lesion in the ipsilateral medial longitudinal fasciculus (MLF)
B. It results in inability to adduct the eye
C. Anterior INO typically preserves convergence
D. Posterior INO is caused by a pontine lesion
E. One-and-a-half syndrome is caused by bilateral MLF lesion and unilateral VI nerve palsy

38.

The following CT was obtained after a car accident. After stabilizing the vital signs, what should be the initial management of the patient?

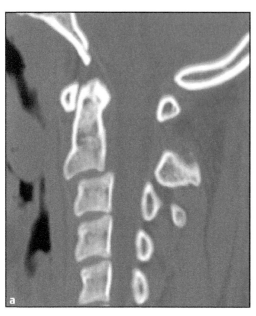

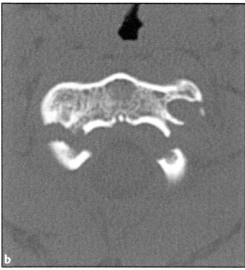

A. Halo immobilization
B. Anterior C2-C3 fusion
C. Posterior C2-C3 fusion
D. Posterior C1-C3 fusion
E. Posterior Occiput-C3 fusion

39.

The syndrome of inappropriate antidiuretic hormone secretion (SIADH) is characterized by all of the following, *except*

A. Hyponatremia
B. Decreased serum osmolarity
C. Decreased serum uric acid
D. Hypovolemia

40.

During a retroperitoneal approach, the nerve that is anterior to the psoas muscle is

A. Obturator n
B. Genitofemoral n
C. Lateral femoral cutaneous n
D. Ilioinguinal n
E. Lumbosacral trunk

41.

Which of the following statements is true about the Hoffmann reflex (H-reflex)?

A. It results from stimulation of the muscle spindle.
B. Afferents travel in Ia fibers.
C. It is produced by supramaximal stimulation.
D. It is a polysynaptic reflex.
E. The latency does *not* depend on the distance between the muscle and the spinal cord.

42.

The following intraparenchymal brain tumor was positive for GFAP (glial fibrillary acid protein) and reticulin. What is the diagnosis?

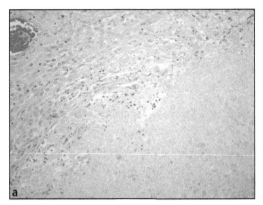

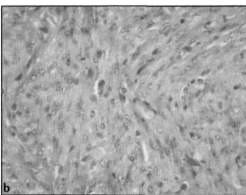

A. Pleomorphic xanthoastrocytoma (PXA)
B. Grade II astrocytoma
C. Grade III astrocytoma
D. Glioblastoma
E. Gliosarcoma

43.

The following is true about Botulinum toxin:

A. Inhibits SNARE (soluble N-ethylmaleimide-sensitive factor-attachment protein-receptor) proteins
B. Competitive muscle blocker
C. Depolarizing muscle blocker
D. Muscarinic receptor blocker
E. Nicotinic receptor ganglion blocker

44.

The following is a radiological sign of occipitocervical dislocation:

A. Powers ratio 1
B. Basion-dens interval (BDI) 13 mm
C. Basion-axis interval (BAI) 11 mm
D. Atlantodental interval (ADI) 6 mm
E. Sun ratio of 2

45.

All of the following is true about neurogenic shock, *except*

A. Hypotension
B. Tachycardia
C. Occurs after spinal cord injury (SCI)
D. Results from autonomic dysfunction
E. Decreased systemic vascular resistance (SVR)

46.

The nucleus responsible for parotid salivary secretion is

A. Nucleus solitarius
B. Nucleus ambiguus
C. Dorsal vagal nucleus
D. Superior salivary nucleus
E. Inferior salivary nucleus

47.

All of the following is true about smooth muscles, *except*

A. They are supplied by autonomic nerves.
B. They have 15 more times actin than myosin.
C. They contain troponin.
D. Contraction is initiated by 4 calcium ions binding calmodulin.
E. Myosin kinase is involved in muscle contraction, while myosin phosphatase in relaxation.

48.

The most common organism recovered from neurosurgical postoperative infection is

A. *Staphylococcus aureus*
B. Group B streptococci
C. *Streptococcus pneumoniae*
D. *Escherichia coli (E. coli)*
E. *Neisseria meningitides*

49.
A 56-year-old female presented with headaches, seizures, and the following MRI. What is the most likely diagnosis?

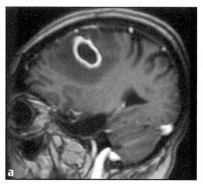 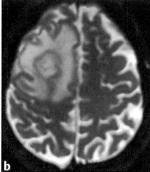 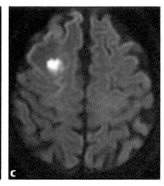

A. Glioblastoma
B. Brain metastasis
C. Multiple sclerosis (MS)
D. Brain abscess

50.
Ramsay Hunt's syndrome is characterized by herpes zoster infection to the

A. Geniculate ganglion
B. Gasserian ganglion
C. Inferior petrosal ganglion
D. Nodose ganglion
E. External auditory canal

51.
Which of the following projections correspond with Mediodorsal (MD)?

A. Areas 18 and 19
B. Area 4
C. Premotor cortex
D. Cingulate gyrus
E. Amygdala

52.
Which of the following projections correspond with Anterior nuclear group (ANG)?

A. Areas 18 and 19
B. Area 4
C. Premotor cortex
D. Cingulate gyrus
E. Amygdala

53.
Which of the following projections correspond with Pulvinar?

A. Areas 18 and 19
B. Area 4
C. Premotor cortex
D. Cingulate gyrus
E. Amygdala

54.
Which of the following projections correspond with Ventral posterolateral, pars oralis (VPLo)?

A. Areas 18 and 19
B. Area 4
C. Premotor cortex
D. Cingulate gyrus
E. Amygdala

55.
Which of the following projections correspond with Ventral lateral, pars oralis (VLo)?

A. Areas 18 and 19
B. Area 4
C. Premotor cortex
D. Cingulate gyrus
E. Amygdala

56.
Which of the following diseases correspond with Bunina bodies?

A. Parkinson's disease
B. Alzheimer's disease
C. Rabies
D. Amyotrophic lateral sclerosis (ALS)
E. Multiple myeloma

57.
Which of the following diseases correspond with Negri bodies?

A. Parkinson's disease
B. Alzheimer's disease
C. Rabies
D. Amyotrophic lateral sclerosis (ALS)
E. Multiple myeloma

58.
Which of the following diseases correspond with Lewy bodies?

A. Parkinson's disease
B. Alzheimer's disease
C. Rabies
D. Amyotrophic lateral sclerosis (ALS)
E. Multiple myeloma

59.
Which of the following diseases correspond with Russel bodies?

A. Parkinson's disease
B. Alzheimer's disease
C. Rabies
D. Amyotrophic lateral sclerosis (ALS)
E. Multiple myeloma

60.
Which of the following diseases correspond with Hirano bodies?

A. Parkinson's disease
B. Alzheimer's disease
C. Rabies
D. Amyotrophic lateral sclerosis (ALS)
E. Multiple myeloma

18 Answer Key 9

1.

C Sarcoidosis

The finding of basilar leptomeningeal enhancement (left frontal) and hilar lymphadenopathy with a sellar/suprasellar mass is highly suggestive of sarcoidosis. ACE (angiotensin-converting enzyme) level should be checked in the serum and/or CSF. Lymph node biopsy via video-assisted cervical mediastinoscopy revealed sarcoidosis.

2.

A Spinal nucleus

The spinal nucleus of the trigeminal nerve (cranial nerve V), pars caudalis is continuous with the substantia gelatinosa of Rolando in the spinal cord and transmits pain, temperature, and crude touch sensations (**Fig. 14**).

3.

E Signals travel through type III and IV fibers

Merkel's discs transmit signals through type II fibers (**Table 2**).

4.

B Basophilic stippling of RBCs (red blood corpuscles)

Basophilic stippling of RBCs is characteristic of lead poisoning. Arsenic poisoning is treated with BAL (British anti-lewisite) (**Table 30**).

5.

D Brain abscesses

The imaging is typical of multiple brain abscesses with a small focus of subdural empyema at the frontal pole. Note the maxillary sinus disease. There is ring-enhancement (**a**), restricted diffusion (brightness) (**b**), and darkness on ADC (**c**). The patient had mucormycosis orbitorhinosinusitis complicated by brain abscesses. He died a week later. Things that are bright on both diffusion and ADC are just T2 shine-through and not diffusion restriction. In tumefactive MS, the ring enhancement is usually incomplete. In GBM and metastases the enhancing wall is usually thicker with irregularities of the inner aspect. Epidermoid cysts have restricted diffusion but are typically located in the cerebellopontine angle and do not enhance.

6.

B Severe cognitive decline

Cognition is typically spared in orbitofrontal syndrome.

Further Reading: Murad A. Le syndrome médiobasal en psychiatrie (Orbitofrontal syndrome in psychiatry). *L'Encéphale*. 1999 Nov-Dec;25(6):634–637

7.

A Lateral femoral cutaneous n

Meralgia paresthetica can complicate iliac crest bone graft harvest from injury to the lateral femoral cutaneous n.

8.

B Hypertension is a known side effect

Main side effects of propofol are respiratory depression and hypotension.

9.

A Alexander's disease

These are all features of Alexander's disease. Macrocephaly is associated with Tay-Sachs disease, Alexander's disease, and Canavan's disease. Rosenthal fibers also occur in pilocytic astrocytoma, but this is a neoplasm not a metabolic disorder (**Table 12**).

10.

C Provides special visceral afferents

The nucleus of tractus solitarius relays taste sensation (special visceral afferents) through cranial nerves VII, IX, and X. General visceral efferents consist of cranial parasympathetic outflow (e.g., salivary nuclei and dorsal vagal nucleus). General somatic efferents include supply to skeletal muscles (e.g., the hypoglossal nucleus), while general somatic afferents include the sensory nuclei of the trigeminal nerve (**Fig. 14**).

11.

C Heparin intravenous (IV) infusion

Females on contraceptive pills are at high risk of sinus thrombosis, especially if dehydrated. CT reveals a spontaneously hyperdense left transverse sinus (**a**) with filling defect with contrast (**b**), sometimes called delta sign. The most important step in treatment is IV heparin, in addition to rehydration. Nimodipine is more appropriate for subarachnoid hemorrhage.

12.

B Spinal accessory n

Injury to the spinal accessory n (cranial nerve XI) is typically seen with lymph node biopsies in the posterior triangle of the neck. The nerve is very superficial in this location. This results in inability to abduct the shoulder beyond 90°, scapular winging, and pain. Suprascapular and axillary nerves do not cause scapular winging. Long thoracic n can give scapular winging and loss of shoulder abduction but the nerve is too deep within the middle scalene muscle and is unlikely to be injured with a lymph node biopsy.

13.

C Blindness

Tolosa–Hunt syndrome is caused by granulomatous inflammation of the lateral wall of the cavernous sinus or superior orbital fissure. It presents typically with painful ophthalmoplegia. It rarely involves the optic n. It is self-limited but can recur. Treatment is with steroids.

14.

D Discitis with epidural abscess

Imaging reveals L5-S1 discitis with epidural abscess. If blood cultures are negative, needle biopsy of the disc should be performed. WBC count, ESR, and CRP should also be checked. If no neurological deficits, treatment is largely conservative with antibiotics and bracing for comfort.

15.

A 14-3-3 protein

The presence of CSF 14-3-3 protein can help establish the diagnosis of sporadic CJD. ACE level is helpful for sarcoidosis, oligoclonal bands for the diagnosis of multiple sclerosis (MS), PLAP for germinomas, and AFP for endodermal sinus tumor and embryonal carcinoma.

16.

A Anterior hypothalamus

Parasympathetic control involves anterior and medial hypothalamus. Sympathetic control: posterior and lateral hypothalamus. Supraoptic and paraventricular nuclei control the release of vasopressin (antidiuretic hormone) and oxytocin, respectively.

17.

E Increased glutamic acid decarboxylase (GAD)

Stiff-man (stiff person, Moersch–Woltman) syndrome is associated with the following antibodies: anti-gephyrin, anti-amphiphysin (paraneoplastic), and anti-GAD (non-paraneoplastic). Phytanic acid oxidase deficiency causes Refsum's disease. Decreased dystrophin is associated with Duchenne's muscular dystrophy. Myophosphorylase deficiency causes McArdle's disease. Anti-Hu antibody is associated with small cell lung cancer and lymphoma; it causes sensory neuropathy involving the dorsal root ganglion (DRG) (**Table 16**).

18.

D Fibrous dysplasia

The ground glass expansion of the skull between 10 and 30 years of age is typical for fibrous dysplasia.

19.

B Hypervolemia

CSWS is associated with hypovolemia (**Table 32**).

20.

B Chordoma

The presence of physaliphorous cells on a mucinous background is a characteristic of chordoma.

21.

E All of the above

Sacral sparing is a sign of incomplete spinal cord injury. Return of the bulbocavernosus reflex means that the patient is not in spinal shock (transient loss of function below the level of the injury) anymore, which makes clinical evaluation more accurate. Testing for sacral sparing includes perianal sensation to pin prick, rectal tone, and plantar flexion of the big toe. It is a good prognostic sign due to the proximity of the spinothalamic tract to the lateral corticospinal tract. In both tracts, the sacral fibers are lateral (**Fig. 15**).

22.

A Sodium-potassium pump

The resting membrane potential is maintained by the sodium-potassium pump; using 1 ATP (adenosine triphosphate), 3 sodium ions go out and 2 potassium ions go in. Rapid sodium influx causes depolarization, potassium efflux causes repolarization, while calcium influx causes neurotransmitter release from presynaptic terminals (**Fig. 27**).

23.

B DNET (dysembryoplastic neuroepithelial tumor)
The presence of large cells (neurons) in mucin, small rounded cells, and chicken-wire vascular pattern are characteristic of DNET. The tumor is common in children, in the temporal lobe, and usually manifests with seizures.

24.

D Medulloblastoma
The highest Cho (cell membrane turnover): NAA (neuronal viability) ratio is found in malignant brain tumors (glioblastoma, medulloblastoma). This is followed by ependymoma, then benign astrocytoma. In normal brain and radiation necrosis, the Cho is almost = NAA.

25.

B B3 (Niacin)
Dementia, diarrhea, and dermatitis (DDD) are symptoms of pellagra, which is associated with vitamin B3 (niacin) deficiency. It is found in predominantly corn eaters. B1 deficiency is associated with beriberi, Wernicke's, and Korsakoff's syndromes. B6 is associated with peripheral neuropathy, B12 with pernicious anemia, and vitamin A with nocturnal blindness.

26.

D Mandibular division of trigeminal n (V_3)
Structures passing through the foramen ovale are V_3, lesser petrosal n, and accessory meningeal a. Cranial n IV passes through the superior orbital fissure outside the annulus of Zinn. V_1 passes through the superior orbital fissure with the lacrimal and frontal branches passing outside the annulus of Zinn while the nasociliary is inside it (remember outside the annulus of Zinn LFT: lacrimal, frontal, and trochlear). V_2 passes through foramen rotundum with the artery of foramen rotundum (from maxillary artery). Middle meningeal a passes through foramen spinosum with the meningeal branch of V_3 (**Fig. 17**).

27.

C Lateral lemniscus
BAER waves: I: cochlear nerve, II: cochlear nuclei, III: superior olivary nucleus, IV: lateral lemniscus, V: inferior colliculus, VI: medial geniculate body, VII: auditory radiation (sublentiform fasciculus) (**Fig. 31**).

28.

A Astrocytic glioma
Li–Fraumeni syndrome is a rare autosomal dominant cancer predisposition syndrome. There is usually p53 mutation on chromosome 17. It is characterized by astrocytic gliomas, soft tissue sarcomas, and breast cancer. Medulloblastoma characterizes the syndromes of Turcot and Gorlin but is rare in Li–Fraumeni. Ependymomas are seen in NF2, but they are rare in Li–Fraumeni. Hemangioblastomas are seen in von Hippel–Lindau disease, while pituitary adenomas are a feature of MEN1 (multiple endocrine neoplasia 1) syndrome (**Table 11**).

Further Reading: Li FP, Fraumeni JF Jr, Mulvihill JJ, et al. A cancer family syndrome in twenty-four kindreds. *Cancer Res.* 1988 Sep 15;48(18):5358–5362

29.

B Autosomal recessive
Huntington's disease inheritance is autosomal dominant, characterized by CAG trinucleotide repeats in IT15 (huntingtin) gene on chromosome 4 (**Table 14**).

Further Reading: Sharp AH, Loev SJ, Schilling G, et al. Widespread expression of Huntington's disease gene (IT15) protein product. *Neuron* 1995 May;14(5):1065–1074

30.

E External rotation
Suprascapular n entrapment is associated with weakness of supraspinatus (shoulder abduction) and infraspinatus (external rotation).

31.

B. Flaccidity
Abrupt intrathecal baclofen withdrawal is an emergency. It is characterized by increased rigidity, fever, seizures, loss of consciousness, labile blood pressure, and hallucination. Untreated, it may lead to rhabdomyolysis, hepatic failure, renal

failure, DIC (disseminated intravascular coagulopathy), and death. The patient should be admitted to the ICU (intensive care unit), oral baclofen started, intravenous (IV) diazepam (Valium) or midazolam (Versed).

Further Reading: Coffey RJ, Edgar TS, Francisco GE, et al. Abrupt withdrawal from intrathecal baclofen: recognition and management of a potentially life-threatening syndrome. *Arch Phys Med Rehabil.* 2002 Jun;83(6):735–741

32.

D It is somatotopically organized with the leg medial.

The lateral spinothalamic tract conveys pain and temperature from the contralateral dorsal horn (layers I, IV, and V) to the VPL of thalamus then the sensory cortex (postcentral gyrus). Somatotopic organization with the leg lateral and the arm medial (**Figs. 8 and 15**).

33.

C Deep peroneal n

The dorsum of the foot is supplied by the superficial peroneal n except the first web space which is supplied by the deep peroneal n. The sural n supplies the lateral aspect of the foot and the little toe. The saphenous n (from the femoral n) supplies the area of the medial malleolus. The tibial nerve supplies the sole of the foot through the medial and lateral plantar nerves and the medial calcaneal branches.

34.

A Choline acetyltransferase

Huntington's disease is associated with choline acetyltransferase deficiency. Acetylcholinesterase inhibition occurs in organophosphate poisoning. Arylsulfatase B deficiency occurs in Maroteaux–Lamy syndrome, sphingomyelinase in Niemann–Pick disease, and iduronate-2-sulfatase in Hunter's disease (**Table 12**).

Further Reading: Aquilonius SM, Eckernäs SA, Sundwall A. Regional distribution of choline acetyltransferase in the human brain: changes in Huntington's chorea. *J Neurol Neurosurg Psychiatr.* 1975 Jul;38(7):669–677

35.

E SEGA (subependymal giant cell astrocytoma)

Note the large astrocytes with large eccentric nuclei. SEGA can be sporadic or occur in tuberous sclerosis. Inheritance of the latter is autosomal dominant on chromosomes 9 or 16.

36.

A Spondylolysis

There is bilateral L5 pars defect: spondylolysis. X-ray also reveals grade I spondylolisthesis (slipped vertebra). Spondyloptosis is a grade V spondylolisthesis where the body of one vertebra drops in front of the body of the vertebra below. Spondylosis means degenerative arthritis of the spine, with development of osteophytes, typically above 40 years old. Ankylosing spondylitis causes bamboo spine and fusion of the facet joints. It is more common in males with HLA-B27 and starts in adolescents and young adults.

37.

C Anterior INO typically preserves convergence.

Convergence is affected in anterior INO (midbrain). Posterior INO is caused by a lesion in the pons and preserves convergence (remember PPP: **P**osterior, **P**ons, **P**reserves convergence).

38.

A Halo immobilization

The initial management of Hangman's fracture should be external immobilization and reduction. Surgery can be considered for Effendi type III fractures (severe angulation with C2-C3 facet dislocation) or failed external immobilization.

39.

D Hypovolemia

SIADH is characterized by normo- or hypervolemia (**Table 32**).

Further Reading: Tisdall M, Crocker M, Watkiss J, Smith M. Disturbances of sodium in critically ill adult neurologic patients: a clinical review. *J Neurosurg Anesthesiol.* 2006 Jan;18(1):57–63

40.

B Genitofemoral n

The lumbar plexus forms inside the psoas major muscle. The genitofemoral n exits anterior to the psoas. Medial to the psoas passes the obturator n, the accessory obturator n, and the lumbosacral trunk. Lateral to the psoas are the iliohypogastric, ilioinguinal, lateral femoral cutaneous, and femoral nn.

41.

B Afferents travel in Ia fibers.

Despite it mimicking the stretch reflex, the H-reflex bypasses the muscle spindle and is obtained by submaximally stimulating the nerve afferents in the Ia fibers. It is a monosynaptic reflex and efferents originate in the alpha motorneuron. The latency increases, the further the muscle is from the spinal cord. The F response is obtained by supramaximal stimulation (**Fig. 27**).

Further Reading: Chen YS, Zhou S. Soleus H-reflex and its relation to static postural control. *Gait Posture* 2011 Feb;33(2):169–178

42.

E Gliosarcoma

Gliosarcoma has two components: glial (**a**) with necrosis, positive for GFAP and sarcoma (**b**) with spindle cells, positive for reticulin.

43.

A Inhibits SNARE (soluble N-ethylmaleimide-sensitive factor-attachment protein-receptor) proteins

Botulinum toxin inhibits SNARE proteins, thus preventing release of acetylcholine from presynaptic terminals. Curare is a competitive muscle blocker, succinylcholine a depolarizing blocker, atropine a muscarinic blocker, and hexamethonium a ganglion blocker (**Figs. 25 and 26**).

44.

B Basion-dens interval (BDI) 13 mm

Radiological signs of occipitocervical dislocation include: Powers ratio >1, BDI (basion to tip of dens) ≥12 mm (Wholey), BAI (basion to posterior axis line) ≥12 mm (Harris), and Sun ratio (C1-C2/C2-C3 interspinous distance) ≥2.5. ADI (back of anterior arch of atlas to front of dens) >3 mm in adults and >5 mm in children is a sign of C1-C2 dislocation.

45.

B Tachycardia

Neurogenic shock occurs after stroke or SCI. It is characterized by loss of sympathetic tone, decreased SVR, hypotension, and bradycardia. Treatment should start with fluid resuscitation. Vasopressors can then be used. Hemorrhagic shock is associated with tachycardia.

46.

E Inferior salivary nucleus

The parasympathetic fibers for parotid secretion originate in the inferior salivary nucleus, travel with the glossopharyngeal n (IX), relay in the otic ganglion then join the auriculotemporal n. The superior salivary nucleus supplies the lacrimal, submandibular, and sublingual glands through cranial nerve VII. The dorsal vagal nucleus supplies parasympathetic to the cardiac, respiratory, and digestive systems. The nucleus *so*li*ta*rius provides *tas*te sensation (VII, IX, and X), while the nucleus ambiguus is special visceral efferent (IX, X, and XI) to palate, pharynx, and larynx (**Fig. 14**).

47.

C They contain troponin.

Smooth muscles have no troponin.

48.

A Staphylococcus aureus

The most common organism recovered from neurosurgical postoperative infections is *Staphylococcus aureus*, *S. epidermidis*, and gram-negative bacilli. *E. coli*, group B streptococci, and listeria monocytogenes are seen in neonates and up to 3 months old. Hemophilus influenza between 3 months and 18 years old, now less common since Hib vaccine. *Neisseria meningitidis* is common in children and young adults (school age). *Streptococcus pneumoniae* is common >50 years old and <3 months old, or after skull base fractures.

49.

D Brain abscess

Although the four options can cause ring enhancement (**a**), in a brain abscess the wall is thin and the inner wall is sharply demarcated. On T2 the hypointense abscess wall contrasts with the hyperintense pus inside and the hyperintense edema outside (**b**). It also shows restricted diffusion (**c**). In MS, the ring is typically incomplete.

50.

A Geniculate ganglion

Ramsay Hunt's syndrome is caused by reactivation of herpes zoster infection to the geniculate ganglion. It causes ear pain, loss of hearing, vertigo, tinnitus, facial weakness, and vesicles in the external ear.

51.

E Amygdala

MD receives afferents from the amygdala, SN, prefrontal cortex, temporal cortex, and GP. It projects to the prefrontal area (**Fig. 8**).

52.

D Cingulate gyrus

ANG receives afferents from the fornix and projects to the cingulate cortex (**Fig. 8**).

53.

A Areas 18 & 19

The pulvinar receives afferents from the superior colliculus and projects to areas 18, 19 (**Fig. 8**).

54.

B Area 4

VPLo and VLc (Vim and Vop) receive afferents from the dentate nucleus and project to motor area 4 (**Fig. 8**).

55.

C Premotor cortex

VLo (Voa) receive afferents from GP and red nucleus and project to the premotor area (**Fig. 8**).

56.

D Amyotrophic lateral sclerosis (ALS)

Bunina bodies are found in anterior horn cells in patients with ALS (**Tables 10** and **13**).

57.

C Rabies

Negri bodies are found in rabies especially in hippocampus (**Table 10**).

58.

A Parkinson's disease

Lewy bodies are found in Parkinson's disease (**Tables 10** and **14**).

59.

E Multiple myeloma

Russel bodies are found in plasma cells in patients with multiple myeloma (**Table 10**).

60.

B Alzheimer's disease

Hirano bodies, neurofibrillary tangles, and neuritic plaques are characteristic of Alzheimer's disease (**Tables 10** and **14**).

19 Test 10—Comprehensive

Yiping Li and Amgad Hanna

1.

Which of the following involuntary movements is seen most commonly after injury to the caudate and putamen?

A. Tremor
B. Hemiballismus
C. Athetosis
D. Dystonia
E. Chorea

2.

Injury to which part of the cerebellum results in dysmetria?

A. Flocculonodular lobe
B. Anterior lobe
C. Interposed nuclei (globose and emboliform)
D. Fastigial nucleus
E. Dentate nucleus

3.

Which of the following symptoms is *not* associated with cluster headache?

A. Female predominance
B. Unilateral
C. Rhinorrhea
D. Sympathetic dysfunction
E. Parasympathetic discharge

4.

Besides the ophthalmic arteries, which other arteries can be thrombosed in temporal arteritis resulting in blindness and ophthalmoplegia?

A. Superficial temporal
B. Facial
C. Vertebral
D. Posterior ciliary
E. Internal maxillary

5.

Which of the following cranial n pain syndromes is associated with syncope and bradycardia?

A. Trigeminal neuralgia
B. Occipital neuralgia
C. Glossopharyngeal neuralgia
D. Hemifacial spasm
E. Ramsay Hunt syndrome

6.

Which vessel is depicted by the arrow in the following cerebral angiogram?

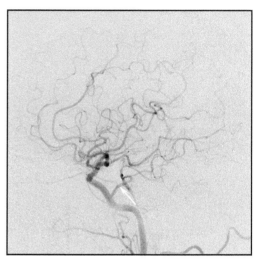

A. Anterior choroidal a
B. PCOM
C. Persistent trigeminal a
D. Hypoglossal a
E. Proatlantal a

7.

A 39-year-old woman presents to the ER after having a transient episode of aphasia and right arm weakness. She recently had fever, joint pain, muscle aches, fatigue, and a malar rash. Antinuclear and anti-Smith antibodies were positive. Which of the following human leukocyte antigen (HLA) alleles is associated with this disease?

A. B47
B. B27
C. DQ2
D. DR3
E. DR4

8.

A 68-year-old man is seen in the clinic with complaints of right-hand weakness. On examination, he has weakness and atrophy of the thenar, hypothenar, and interossei as well as decreased sensation on the ulnar aspect of the hand. Compound muscle action potentials are decreased for the median and ulnar nerves while sensory latencies are prolonged for the ulnar n only. The constellation of clinical features is characteristic of which neurologic pattern?

A. Wartenberg's sign
B. Gilliatt–Sumner hand
C. Froment's sign
D. Jeanne's sign
E. Gamekeeper's sign

9.

A 29-year-old woman presents with a 6-month history of relapsing and remitting difficulties with gait, muscle weakness, and double vision. On examination, she has nystagmus, intention tremor, and scanning speech. Which of the following evoked potentials are most useful for diagnosis?

A. Brainstem auditory evoked potentials
B. Somatosensory evoked potentials
C. Visual evoked potentials
D. Motor evoked potentials
E. Laser evoked potentials

10.

Stimulation of which gaze center results in ipsilateral horizontal conjugate eye movements?

A. Superior colliculus
B. Inferior colliculus
C. Rostral interstitial nucleus (riMLF)
D. Paramedian pontine reticular formation (PPRF)
E. Frontal eye fields

11.

Which of the following eye movements present rhythmically with the same speed in both directions and are associated with head nodding in infants?

A. See-saw nystagmus
B. Convergence nystagmus
C. Downbeat nystagmus
D. Ocular bobbing
E. Spasmus nutans

12.

An 8-year-old boy has been frequently sent to detention by the teacher because of failure to answer questions when prompted in class. The teacher notes the student is unresponsive when addressed and acts weird when he does respond. He will often stare blankly into space instead of paying attention in class. If you suspect a seizure disorder, which anticonvulsant is the first-line treatment?

A. Carbamazepine
B. Phenytoin
C. Levetiracetam
D. Phenobarbital
E. Ethosuximide

13.

Which of the following anticonvulsants has the longest half-life?

A. Carbamazepine
B. Phenytoin
C. Levetiracetam
D. Phenobarbital
E. Ethosuximide

14.

Which of the following will result in mid-sized fixed pupils?

A. Third cranial n palsy
B. Pontine lesion
C. Death
D. Atropine toxicity
E. Opiates

15.

A 5-year-old boy is being evaluated for sleepwalking. He frequently wakes up with bruises on his knees and elbows. During which stage of sleep does this typically occur?

A. REM
B. Stage 4 and REM
C. Stage 3 and 4
D. Stage 2
E. Stage 1

16.

A 65-year-old man undergoes emergent endovascular thrombectomy and thrombolysis for an acute basilar a thrombosis. Postoperatively he was found to have bilateral parieto-occipital cortical infarcts but makes a good recovery. On examination, he is unable to look voluntarily at a peripheral field while his extraocular muscle function is intact during involuntary gaze. He has difficulty fixating the eyes and is unable to move his hand to a specific object using vision. Which syndrome is he likely to be suffering from?

A. Balint's syndrome
B. Disconnection syndrome
C. Gerstmann's syndrome
D. Anton's syndrome
E. Claude's syndrome

17.

A 64-year-old female presents with speech difficulty and memory problems. She has a history of anal squamous cell carcinoma. She does not smoke and does not drink alcohol. On examination, she has expressive aphasia. MRI is shown below. Left temporal open biopsy was performed, the histology is shown below. What is the diagnosis?

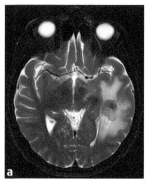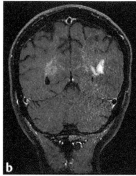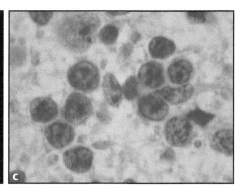

A. Toxoplasmosis
B. Lymphoma
C. Gliomatosis cerebri
D. Herpes encephalitis
E. Progressive multifocal leukoencephalopathy (PML)

18.
Which of the following enzymes is responsible for catalyzing the conversion of L-DOPA to dopamine?

A. Aldehyde dehydrogenase
B. Monoamine oxidase
C. Phenylalanine hydroxylase
D. Tyrosine hydroxylase
E. Tryptophan decarboxylase

19.
A 21-year-old man presents with progressive myelopathy. MRI of the cervical spine reveals a ventral cystic intradural extramedullary mass. You suspect a neurenteric cyst. What is the origin of this type of lesion?

A. Neural crest
B. Notochord
C. Endoderm
D. Mesoderm
E. Ectoderm

20.
Which of the following is *not* characteristic of cisplatin toxicity?

A. Nephrotoxicity
B. Leukoencephalopathy
C. Ototoxicity
D. Visual loss
E. Nausea and Vomiting

21.
A 5-month old infant presents with an abnormally shaped head. The parents note he is developing normally and had an uncomplicated delivery. On examination, he has scaphocephaly (boat-shaped head). Which of the following is associated with the development of secondary sagittal craniosynostosis?

A. Rickets
B. Vitamin A deficiency
C. Hypothyroidism
D. Hyperphosphatemia
E. Hypercortisolemia

22.
Carotid sinus and body input are transmitted through which of the following?

A. Scarpa's ganglion
B. Petrosal ganglion
C. Superior ganglion of cranial n IX
D. Nodosal ganglion
E. Jugular ganglion

23.
Parasympathetic input to the genitals, bowel, and bladder is transmitted through which nerves?

A. Nervi erigentes
B. Hypogastric plexus
C. Pudendal n
D. Genitofemoral n
E. Iliohypogastric n

24.
Localization of sound is regulated by which of the following structures?

A. Inferior colliculus
B. Superior olivary nucleus
C. Lateral lemniscus
D. Medial geniculate body
E. Heschl's gyrus

25.
While performing a retrosigmoid craniotomy for a cerebellopontine angle mass, you lose wave V of the brainstem auditory evoked potentials. What anatomic structures does this correlate with?

A. Cochlea
B. Superior olive
C. Lateral lemniscus
D. Inferior colliculus
E. Medial geniculate body

26.
Which of the following is *false* regarding Renshaw cells?

A. Renshaw cells are found in the anterior horn of the spinal cord
B. They use the neurotransmitter glycine
C. They inhibit surrounding α-motor neuron agonists
D. They inhibit surrounding α-motor neuron antagonists
E. They create a negative feedback loop on multiple motor neurons

27.
Which of the following is *false* regarding muscle spindles?

A. The muscle stretch reflex is a polysynaptic reflex
B. Muscle spindles are in parallel with muscle fibers
C. They detect both length and velocity of change in length of the muscle fibers
D. They contain both type Ia and type II nerve fibers
E. The muscle spindle output is sensory

28.

A 74-year-old male with a history of hypertension, type 2 diabetes mellitus, and stroke presents with acute onset of left-sided hemiparesis, neglect, and right-sided gaze deviation. A hyperdense MCA sign is found on CT scan consistent with a thrombus in the proximal M1 segment. Which Brodmann area results in contralateral gaze deviation after an infarction?

A. Brodmann's area 2
B. Brodmann's area 4
C. Brodmann's area 6
D. Brodmann's area 8
E. Brodmann's area 10

29.

A 36-year-old female has been suffering from epilepsy since childhood. She presents for a surgical opinion after video-EEG localizes seizures to bilateral amygdala. She undergoes gross total resection of bilateral amygdala while sparing the hippocampi. Postoperatively she develops Klüver–Bucy syndrome. Which collection of symptoms is *not* part of this syndrome?

A. Increased sex drive (hypersexuality)
B. Decreased aggressiveness (docility)
C. Visual agnosia
D. Hypophagia
E. Forgetfulness (amnesia)

30.

Which of the following is true regarding slow-wave sleep?

A. Stage 1 sleep is associated with low-voltage high-frequency β waves
B. Stage 2 sleep is characterized by sleep spindles and K complexes
C. Stage 3 sleep is characterized by β waves
D. Stage 4 sleep is characterized by θ waves
E. None of the above

31.

Which of the following is *false* regarding spinal muscular atrophy type 1 (Werdnig–Hoffmann disease)?

A. It is the most common form of spinal muscular atrophy
B. It has autosomal dominant inheritance
C. The responsible gene is found on chromosome 5q
D. Onset is during infancy
E. There is no associated mental retardation

32.

A 68-year-old male hospitalized with an acute right MCA stroke develops malignant cerebral edema and dies 4 days later. At autopsy, what is the most likely finding?

A. Hyperchromatic cells, red swollen neurons, and edema
B. Accumulation of polymorphonuclear leukocytes (PMNs)
C. Peak concentration of PMNs
D. Accumulation of macrophages
E. Development of neovascularization

33.

You are consulted on a 1-week-old, 32-week premature infant after the pediatrician noticed a dramatically increasing head circumference. A cranial ultrasound was performed and revealed a large intraparenchymal hemorrhage in the right basal ganglia with extension of the hemorrhage into the insula and the ventricle with associated hydrocephalus. What grade of germinal matrix bleeding is it?

A. Grade 1
B. Grade 2
C. Grade 3
D. Grade 4
E. Grade 5

34.

A 62-year-old male is brought to the ER for ataxia, slurred speech, and cognitive changes. The patient has a history of hypertension, type 2 diabetes mellitus, and renal failure. He does not smoke cigarettes, but consumes four alcoholic drinks per week. On examination, he was noticed to have dysarthria, nystagmus, dysmetria, myoclonus, and ataxic gait. Diffusion-weighted MRI is shown below. The patient's mental status continued to deteriorate rapidly and he succumbed to his disease after 5 days. Brain autopsy findings are shown below. What is the most likely diagnosis?

A. Ischemic stroke
B. Lymphoma
C. Prion disease
D. Wernicke's encephalopathy
E. Hypertensive encephalopathy

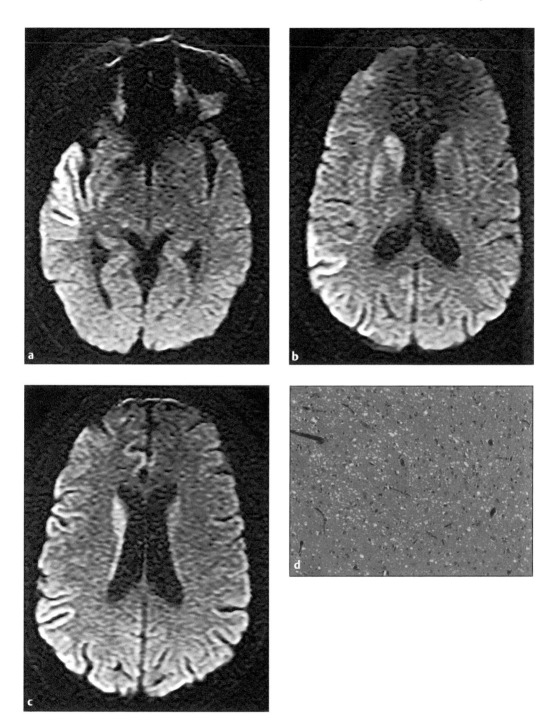

35.

The following picture was taken intra-operatively during an endoscopic third ventriculostomy. What anatomic structure represents the fornix?

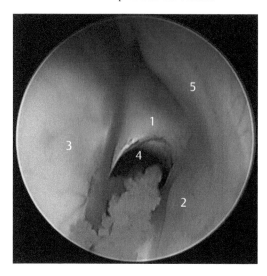

A. 1
B. 2
C. 3
D. 4
E. 5

36.

In the same figure, the caudate nucleus is represented by

A. 1
B. 2
C. 3
D. 4
E. 5

37.

The following picture was taken intra-operatively during an endoscopic third ventriculostomy. The location of the third ventriculostomy (*arrow*) is in the

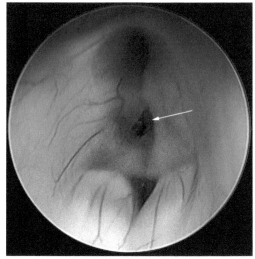

A. Tuber cinereum
B. Basilar artery
C. Mammillary bodies
D. Infundibular recess
E. Chiasmatic recess

38.

The following picture was taken intra-operatively during an endoscopic third ventriculostomy. What anatomic structure is marked by the *arrow*?

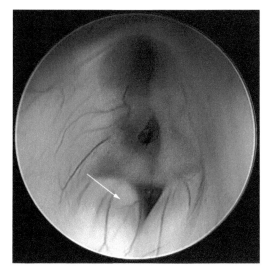

A. Tuber cinereum
B. Basilar artery
C. Mammillary bodies
D. Infundibular recess
E. Chiasmatic recess

39.
A 24-year-old male presents with headache and diplopia. MRI is shown below. Upon removal of the tumor, the following histology was revealed. What is the diagnosis?

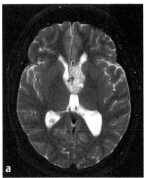
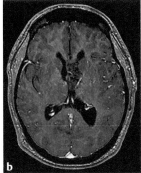
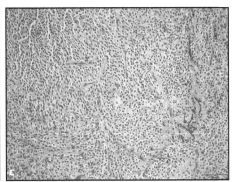

A. SEGA
B. Subependymoma
C. Ependymoma
D. PNET
E. Central neurocytoma

40.
A 19-year-old male presents to the ER after being involved in a motorcycle accident. He complains of neck pain, decreased sensation and numbness and tingling in the fingers, as well as burning in the hands. On examination, he has grade 4 motor strength in the upper extremities proximally and grade 2 distally. The lower extremities and cranial nerves are intact. What syndrome does this patient have?

A. Brown–Séquard syndrome
B. Wallenberg's syndrome
C. Anterior cord syndrome
D. Posterior cord syndrome
E. Central cord syndrome

41.
A 78-year-old man has a known diagnosis of small cell lung cancer and has been complaining of weakness especially involving the muscles of the proximal arms and legs. His strength improves throughout the day. Which of the following is *false* regarding Lambert–Eaton myasthenic syndrome?

A. Antibodies develop against presynaptic VGCC
B. There is a decrease in Ach release from the presynaptic terminal
C. It spares the autonomic nervous system
D. There is an incremental response on EMG
E. LEMS affects males predominantly

42.
Duchenne's muscular dystrophy and Becker's muscular dystrophy share many of the same characteristics, *except* which of the following?

A. X-linked recessive
B. Calf pseudohypertrophy
C. Commonly present with mental retardation
D. Positive Gower's test
E. Weakness involves pelvic muscles

43.
During an EMG, which of the following correlates with a direct motor response caused by stimulation of a motor nerve?

A. H-reflex
B. M wave
C. F wave
D. Fibrillation
E. Fasciculation

44.

Which of the following is *not* a sign of reinnervation on EMG?

A. Decreased amplitude
B. Polyphasic units
C. Fibrillation potentials
D. Formation of giant units
E. None of the above

45.

Which of the following is *false* regarding resistance to passive movement in spasticity?

A. Bidirectional
B. Velocity dependent
C. Increased deep tendon reflexes
D. Clasp knife
E. Clonus

46.

A 28-year-old Asian woman presents to the ER with transient episodes of aphasia. A non-contrast head CT is negative. Based on the following angiogram findings, what associated disease could worsen the patient's prognosis?

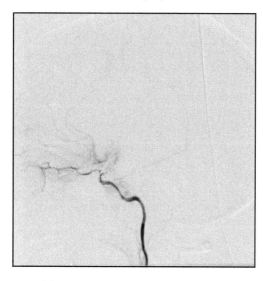

A. Diabetes
B. Hypertension
C. Grave's disease
D. Polycystic kidney disease
E. Hypercholesterolemia

47.

A 16-year-old girl presents with a two-day history of severe headaches associated with nausea and vomiting, and now complains of diplopia. The only medications she takes is for birth control. MR venogram is shown below. The most likely associated cranial nerve palsy is

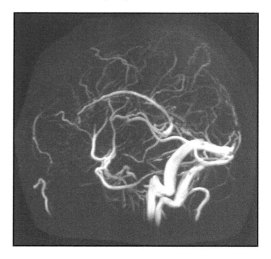

A. Oculomotor n
B. Trigeminal n
C. Abducens n
D. Vagus n
E. Hypoglossal n

48.

A 43-year-old male presents with a first-time seizure. While watching television, he started complaining of epigastric discomfort then lost consciousness and fell off his chair. He was taken to the ER where a dilated right pupil was noted. A non-contrast head CT which was performed is shown below. What is the most likely diagnosis?

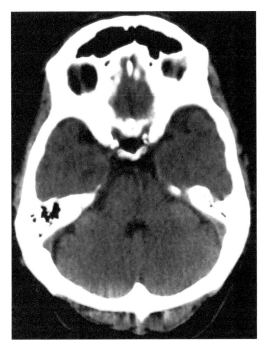

A.   PCOM aneurysm
B.   Limbic encephalitis
C.   Cavernous malformation
D.   Contusion
E.   Temporal glioma

49.

A 33-year-old woman presents with a one-year history of back pain, pain radiating down the left buttock and the left leg. An MRI of the lumbar spine were performed. What is the most likely histologic finding of a tumor in this region?

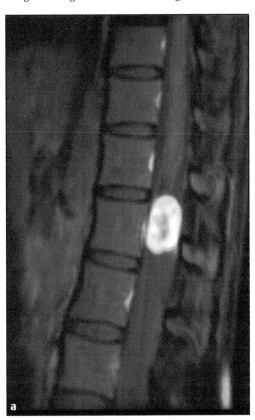

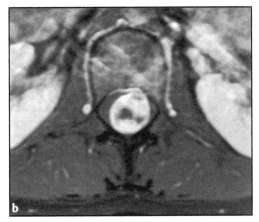

A.   Verocay bodies
B.   Rosenthal fibers
C.   Mitosis and necrosis
D.   Well-differentiated cuboidal cells radially oriented around myxoid cores
E.   Dilated vessels with thin walls

50.

A 3-month-old infant presents with a scalp mass. On examination, it is red, non-tender, but soft and fluctuant and on palpation there appears to be a bony defect surrounding this lesion. There is no evidence of a dimple or cutaneous tract. An MRI is performed. What is the diagnosis?

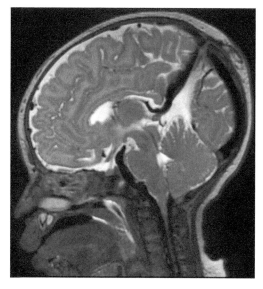

A. Epidermoid cyst
B. Eosinophilic granuloma
C. Dermal sinus tract
D. Sinus pericranii
E. Atretic cephalocele

51.

The parents of a 7-year-old girl note the patient has been increasingly clumsy over the past few months. She has been running into the furniture while walking and has multiple bruises on her right side. On examination, she has over 10 pigmented, flat spots on various areas of the skin. In addition to the lesion shown in the MRI, what is an additional major criterion to confirm the diagnosis?

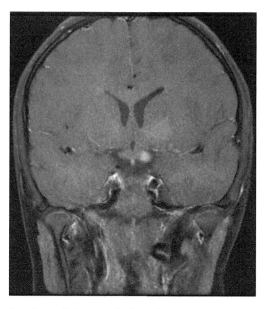

A. Second-degree relative with NF1
B. First-degree relative with NF2
C. One plexiform neurofibroma
D. One Lisch nodule
E. Three café-au-lait spots

52.
A 4-year-old girl presents to the ER after being involved in a high-speed motor vehicle accident. She complains of neck pain but is otherwise neurologically intact. The following image was obtained, which shows a synchondrosis fracture of the axis. How many primary ossification centers are normally seen in the axis?

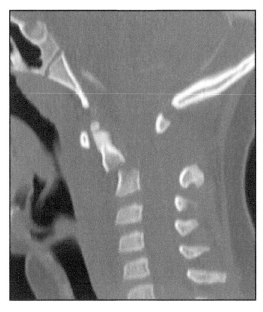

A. 1
B. 2
C. 3
D. 4
E. 5

53.
A 24-year-old man is brought to the ER with a fever of 103°F, shortness of breath, and a 3-week history of back pain. On examination, he has tenderness to palpation in the mid lumbar spine and bilateral consolidations on chest X-ray. Additional imaging studies confirm discitis with osteomyelitis. His ABG shows a pH of 7.18, $PaCO_2$ of 68 mmHg, and PaO_2 of 55 mmHg. His serum Na is 138 mEq/L, K 4.2 mEq/L, Cl 102 mEq/L, and HCO_3 of 24 mEq/L. Which of the following is true?

A. The patient has a respiratory acidosis
B. The patient has a mixed respiratory and metabolic acidosis
C. The patient has an anion gap acidosis
D. The patient has a respiratory alkalosis
E. The patient has a respiratory acidosis with compensatory metabolic alkalosis

54.
A 55-year-old man is admitted to the ICU with decreased level of consciousness and Kussmaul respirations. He localizes to noxious stimulation and becomes irritable with cares. His mucous membranes are dry and eyes are sunken. His laboratory studies show Na 126 mEq/L, K 4.8 mEq/L, Cl 100 mEq/L, Glucose 1100 mg/dL. What is his corrected sodium based on these results?

A. 121 mEq/L
B. 126 mEq/L
C. 131 mEq/L
D. 136 mEq/L
E. 142 mEq/L

55.
Which of the following is true regarding the absolute refractory period of a neuronal action potential?

A. Sodium channels remain open
B. Potassium channels remain open
C. The neuron will fire with a supra normal stimulus
D. Calcium channels are the main regulators of repolarization
E. Membrane stabilizers such as local anesthetics can overcome the absolute refractory period

56.
Which of the following is *false* regarding the neuron membrane potential?

A. The axonal resting membrane potential is −90 mV
B. Depolarization is a result of opening of Na channels
C. Cl⁻ permeability does *not* greatly contribute to the action potential
D. The action potential of a neuron starts at the axon hillock
E. An action potential can only be initiated once the resting potential reaches −25 mV

57.

Which of the following cortical cell layer(s) send efferent signals to the brain stem and spinal cord?

A.   Layer I

B.   Layer II and III

C.   Layer IV

D.   Layer V

E.   Layer VI

58.

Which neurotransmitter is secreted by the neurons of the periaqueductal gray and periventricular hypothalamus and is involved in pain inhibition and analgesia?

A.   Acetylcholine

B.   Serotonin

C.   Dopamine

D.   Glycine

E.   Glutamate

59.

Fast pain fibers (Aδ) enter the spinal cord through Lissauer's tract posterior to the dorsal horn before terminating in which Rexed lamina?

A.   Lamina I (marginal nucleus)

B.   Lamina II (substantia gelatinosa of Rolando)

C.   Lamina III (nucleus proprius)

D.   Lamina VII (intermediolateral nucleus)

E.   Lamina IX (Onuf's nucleus)

60.

A three-year-old boy presents with increased irritability, abdominal pain, ataxia, and new onset seizures. He is noted to have gingival lead line on examination on his oral mucosa and plumbism is suspected. Which laboratory study is most consistent with the diagnosis?

A.   Megaloblastic anemia

B.   Increased urine lead levels

C.   Increased urine coproporphyrin III

D.   Decreased serum aminolevulinic acid levels

E.   Increased serum total iron binding capacity (TIBC)

20 Answer Key 10

Yiping Li and Amgad Hanna

1.

E Chorea

Chorea is a brisk arrhythmic movement associated with *H*untington's disease, rheumatic *h*eart disease, and *h*aloperidol (3Hs). It can be associated with *h*ypotonia and pendular reflexes. Hemiballismus is due to a lesion in the contralateral STN, athetosis in the globus pallidus, and Parkinson's disease in SN (**Fig. 7**).

2.

E Dentate nucleus

The flocculonodular lobe (archicerebellum) is involved with equilibrium and nystagmus. Injury to the fastigial nucleus (vermis) results in truncal ataxia (inability to sit, stand, or walk) and scanning speech. Injury to the anterior lobe (paleocerebellum) disrupts spinocerebellar tracts from muscle tendons. This connects with the interposed nuclei and functions with muscle tone and posture, thereby resulting in increased extensor tone (in dogs) and gait ataxia (tandem walk—heel-to-toe test) when injured. The dentate nucleus (neocerebellum) input is corticopontine, it connects with the cerebellar hemispheres (posterior lobe), and injury causes intention tremor, ipsilateral ipsilateral dysmetria (finger-to-nose test), dysarthria, hypotonia, and poor voluntary movement planning and coordination (dysdiadokokinesia: inability to perform rapid alternating movements).

3.

A Female predominance

Unlike most other types of headache, cluster headache has a male predominance.

4.

D Posterior ciliary

In temporal arteritis, thrombosis of the posterior ciliary and ophthalmic aa is associated with amaurosis fugax and ophthalmoplegia due to granulomatous inflammation. Giant cells are seen on temporal a biopsy and patients typically present with temporal headaches, jaw pain, and shoulder pain. Treatment includes corticosteroids until ESR normalizes (**Table 29**).

5.

C Glossopharyngeal neuralgia

Glossopharyngeal neuralgia is characterized by pain in the tonsillar fossa elicited by swallowing and is associated with bradycardia and syncope due to irritation and stimulation of the nerve of the carotid body and sinus (Hering's n).

6.

C Persistent trigeminal a

Persistent trigeminal a (*arrow*) connects the ICA anteriorly (precavernous or proximal cavernous) to the basilar a posteriorly. It is observed in 0.1–0.5% of cerebral angiograms.

7.

D DR3

Systemic lupus erythematosus is associated with DR2 and 3. Ankylosing spondylitis is associated with the HLA-B27 allele. Congenital adrenal hyperplasia (21-hydroxylase deficiency) with B47, celiac disease with DQ2, Sjogren's syndrome with DR3, and rheumatoid arthritis with DR4.

8.

B Gilliatt–Sumner hand

Gilliatt–Sumner hand is seen in neurogenic thoracic outlet syndrome with involvement of the lower trunk of the brachial plexus. There is involvement of the median and ulnar motor with ulnar sensory both clinically and by EMG/NCS. Wartenberg's, Jeanne's (hyperextension of the metacarpophalangeal joint with flexion of the interphalangeal joint of the thumb), and Froment's signs are tests for ulnar nerve weakness whereas Gamekeeper's is a test for ulnar collateral ligament tears at the thumb.

9.

C Visual evoked potentials

Visual evoked potentials are the most useful in the diagnosis of multiple sclerosis; they identify impaired transmission along the optic pathways which is an early finding in MS.

10.

D Paramedian pontine reticular formation (PPRF)

PPRF stimulates the ipsilateral VI n and contralateral III n. Stimulation of the frontal eye fields or the superior colliculus results in contralateral horizontal conjugate gaze. The riMLF is the vertical gaze center.

11.

E Spasmus nutans

Spasmus nutans occurs in the first 2 years of life and is characterized by ocular oscillations, head nodding, and abnormal head position. See-saw nystagmus is seen with parasellar lesions, convergence nystagmus is caused by includes pineal lesions, downbeat nystagmus is caused by cervicomedullary junction tumors, and ocular bobbing is seen with pontine masses.

12.

E Ethosuximide

Ethosuximide and valproic acid are first-line medications to treat absence seizures (**Table 34**).

13.

D Phenobarbital

Side effects of phenobarbital can be lethargy and nystagmus. The half-life is 96 hours which is the longest out of all the anticonvulsants. Valproic acid has the shortest half-life of 8 hours (**Table 34**).

14.

C Death

Brain death is associated with mid-size fixed pupils due to loss of both sympathetic and parasympathetic output to the eye. Atropine and III n palsy result in fixed and dilated pupils, while pontine lesions and opiates result in pinpoint pupils.

15.

C Stage 3 and 4

Sleepwalking (somnambulism) and night terrors occur during stage 3 or 4 sleep, nightmares occur during REM sleep, and nocturnal epilepsy occurs in stage 4 and REM (**Fig. 31**).

16.

A Balint's syndrome

Balint's syndrome is a rare manifestation of parietal lobe lesions. It manifests with optic ataxia (inability to move the hand toward an object that is seen), oculomotor apraxia (difficulty fixating the eyes), and simultagnosia (inability to perceive more than one object at a time in the visual field). Disconnection syndrome presents with apraxia of the left hand. Gerstmann's syndrome is characterized by agraphia, acalculia, finger agnosia, and left–right dissociation. Anton's syndrome (also called Anton–Babinski) is cortical blindness (visual anosognosia) with denial due to lesions of bilateral occipital lobes. Claude's syndrome is oculomotor palsy with contralateral ataxia due to a midbrain lesion.

17.

B Lymphoma

Pathology shows loosely arranged B-lymphocytes with prominent nucleoli confirming the diagnosis of lymphoma. Note the multiple periventricular lesions on MRI: left temporal (**a**) (the one biopsied) and bilateral on coronal (**b**).

18.

E Tryptophan decarboxylase

Tryptophan decarboxylase (also known as DOPA decarboxylase or aromatic L-aminoacid decarboxylase) converts L-DOPA to dopamine. Tyrosine hydroxylase converts tyrosine to L-DOPA and is the first and rate-limiting step.

19.

C Endoderm

Neurenteric cysts are composed of heterotopic endodermal tissue. Histopathology reveals columnar or cuboidal epithelium characteristic of respiratory or gastrointestinal tissue. These are benign lesions.

20.

B Leukoencephalopathy

Subacute necrotizing leukoencephalitis (SNLE) is frequently seen in methotrexate toxicity whereas cisplatin affects microtubules and typically involves the peripheral nervous system (**Table 30**).

21.

A Rickets

Vitamin D deficiency (rickets), hyperthyroidism, hypophosphatemia, and sickle cell disease are associated with secondary craniosynostosis.

22.

B Petrosal ganglion

The petrosal (inferior) ganglion of IX receives taste and carotid sinus and body (Hering's n) input. The superior ganglion of IX as well as superior (jugular) ganglion of X receive ear sensation. The nodose (inferior) ganglion of X controls taste and visceral sensation. Scarpa's ganglion encompasses the superior and inferior vestibular ganglia and controls vestibular function with the utricle to the superior ganglion and saccule to the inferior ganglion.

23.

A Nervi erigentes

The pelvic splanchnic nn (nervi erigentes) are the preganglionic parasympathetic fibers from S2, S3, and S4 to the pelvic organs and hindgut. The hypogastric plexus (superior and inferior) provides sympathetic input while the pudendal, genitofemoral, and iliohypogastric nn are somatic.

24.

B Superior olivary nucleus

Sound localization is achieved by the superior olivary nucleus where the **m**edial nuclei detect the ti**m**e lag between the ears while the lateral ones detect the difference in intensity.

25.

D Inferior colliculus

The mnemonic ECOLI MR can be used for the anatomical correlations of BAER waves, with wave I corresponding to the **E**ighth nerve, II **C**ochlear nuclei, III superior **O**live, IV **L**ateral Lemniscus, V **I**nferior colliculus, VI **M**edial geniculate body, and VII auditory **R**adiation (**Fig. 31**).

26.

D They inhibit surrounding a-motor neuron antagonists.

Renshaw cells are primarily inhibitory interneurons found in the gray matter of the spinal cord. They receive excitatory input from the α-motor neuron and inhibit the α-motor neurons within the same group (agonists), thereby creating a negative feedback. They inhibit the inhibitory interneurons, resulting in stimulation of the antagonists (**Fig. 27**). They utilize the neurotransmitter glycine which causes Cl⁻ influx.

27.

A The muscle stretch reflex is a polysynaptic reflex.

The muscle spindle is found in the belly of skeletal muscles and detects changes in length of muscle fibers. It is stimulated when stretched and the impulses travel through Ia fibers to α-motor neurons that cause contraction through a monosynaptic reflex (**Fig. 28**).

28.

D Brodmann's area 8

The frontal eye fields correspond to Brodmann's area 8. Area 2 is the primary sensory cortex, area 4 is the primary motor cortex, area 6 is the supplementary motor area, and area 10 is the prefrontal cortex (**Figs. 1 and 2**).

29.

D Hypophagia

In Klüver–Bucy syndrome, patients will often have increased appetite and eat uncontrollably especially eating inappropriate objects (pica). This syndrome is seen in bilateral lesions of the medial temporal lobe.

30.

B Stage 2 sleep is characterized by sleep spindles and K complexes.

Stage 1 sleep is characterized by low-voltage low-frequency α waves. β waves are associated with awake alert state and REM sleep. Stage 2 sleep is characterized by sleep spindles and K complexes while stages 3 and 4 are characterized by delta waves (>50% in stage 4) (**Fig. 31**).

31.

B It has autosomal dominant inheritance.

Werdnig–Hoffmann disease is the most common and worst form of SMA and is inherited in an autosomal recessive pattern on chromosome 5q. It affects the tongue, proximal extensor, and trunk muscles (**Table 13**).

32.

D Accumulation of macrophages

At 6 hours after an infarct, the neurons are hyperchromatic and cerebral edema develops. By 24 hours the introduction of PMNs occurs and peaks after 48 hours. By 3–5 days macrophages arrive and continue to accumulate until neovascularization occurs after 2 weeks.

33.

D Grade 4

Grade 1 is limited to the germinal matrix, grade 2 involves the ventricle without hydrocephalus, grade 3 has hydrocephalus, and grade 4 has intraparenchymal hemorrhage. There is no grade 5 germinal matrix bleeding.

34.

C Prion disease

The patient has subacute spongiform encephalopathy (Prion disease, Creutzfeldt–Jakob disease, CJD). Typical clinical findings are rapidly progressive dementia, myoclonus, and ataxia. Diffusion-weighted MRI revealed cortical ribboning in the right temporoparietal cortex (**a, b, c**) and diffusion restriction in the right corpus striatum (**b, c**). Involvement of the dorsomedial thalamus and pulvinar can give the hockey-stick sign. Gross autopsy can reveal brain atrophy. Histology shows vacuoles (**d**) (spongiform changes). Work-up can include EEG, typically showing periodic sharp wave complexes. CSF findings include 14-3-3 protein and RT-QuIC.

35.

A 1

Fornix (1) forms the superior and anterior border of the foramen of Monro (4). The choroid plexus lies between the thalamus (2) laterally and the septum pellucidum (3) medially. The latter has the septal v coursing anteriorly from the foramen of Monro (**Figs. 22 and 23**).

36.

E 5

The caudate nucleus (5) is lateral to the thalamus (2). Septum pellucidum is medial to the choroid plexus and can be identified with the septal v (**Figs. 22 and 23**).

37.

A Tuber cinereum

The tuber cinereum of the hypothalamus is the site of a third ventriculostomy which lies between the mammillary bodies and the infundibular recess (**Fig. 23B**).

38.

C Mammillary bodies

The mammillary bodies are identified on either side just posterior to the tuber cinereum which is the site of third ventriculostomy (**Fig. 23B**).

39.

E Central neurocytoma

Central neurocytoma occurs in the lateral ventricles of young adults (20 to 40 years old) and variably enhances with gadolinium, in this case there is mild heterogeneous enhancement. It consists of small round cells, sometimes with halos similar to oligodendrogliomas. They are immunoreactive to synaptophysin and electron microscopy reveals vesicles.

40.

E Central cord syndrome

Central cord syndrome predominantly involves the hands due to their medial location in the corticospinal and spinothalamic tracts (**Fig. 15**). Brown–Séquard syndrome presents with decreased contralateral pain and temperature sensation and ipsilateral proprioception loss with weakness. Anterior spinal cord (Beck's) syndrome results in bilateral hypesthesia due to loss of the spinothalamic tract and spastic paralysis due to injury to the corticospinal tracts. Posterior cord involves the dorsal columns and presents with reduced proprioception. Wallenberg's syndrome involves the lateral medulla (**Fig. 13**).

41.

C It spares the autonomic nervous system.

Lambert–Eaton myasthenic syndrome involves the autonomic nervous system but spares the ocular and bulbar muscles and is seen most commonly with small cell lung cancer. It is caused by antibodies against presynaptic VGCC (**Fig. 26**). There is no response to anticholinesterase medications. EMG shows incremental response if high-frequency stimulation (>20 Hz), but decremental at low-frequency stimulation (2–5 Hz). In myasthenia gravis, response is decremental.

42.

C Commonly present with mental retardation

Mental retardation is rarely seen in Becker's muscular dystrophy. In Duchenne's muscular dystrophy, there is decreased dystrophin in contrast to normal levels of abnormally functioning dystrophin in Becker's (**Table 13**).

Further Reading: Ho R, Nguyen ML, Mather P. Cardiomyopathy in Becker muscular dystrophy: overview. *World J Cardiol.* 2016;8(6):356–361

43.

B M wave

M wave is a direct motor response that does not pass through the spinal cord (fastest). H-reflex is elicited by a submaximal stimulation of a sensory fiber (Ia), which in turn activates a motor neuron. It is the electrical equivalent of the muscle stretch reflex. F response is the supramaximal stimulation of a motor or a mixed nerve resulting in retrograde and subsequent anterograde impulses to the muscle through the α-motor neuron resulting in a contraction (**Fig. 27**). Fibrillation and fasciculation are spontaneous activities.

44.

C Fibrillation potentials

Fibrillation potentials are spontaneous depolarizations observed with muscle denervation and probably correlate with Wallerian degeneration. Nascent potentials are small, polyphasic, and represent a true sign of axonal regeneration. Polyphasic units result from terminal collateral sprouting (early, ~2 mo). Giant units are >8 mV and result from the summation of multiple motor units; they are usually a sign of chronicity (yrs, e.g., poliomyelitis).

45.

A Bidirectional

Spasticity is a manifestation of upper motor neuron lesion with reduced inhibition of α-motor neurons (**Fig. 28**). It is unidirectional. In contrast, rigidity (seen in extrapyramidal lesions, like Parkinson's disease) is bidirectional, velocity independent, lead pipe or cog wheel, with normal deep tendon reflexes, and with no clonus.

Further Reading: Mukherjee A, Chakravarty A. Spasticity mechanisms—for the clinician. *Front Neurol.* 2010 Dec 17;1:149

46.

C Grave's disease

Graves' disease with thyrotoxicosis can be associated with Moyamoya disease (shown here on the angiogram) and precipitate cerebral ischemic events. Thyroid hormones may augment vascular sensitivity to sympathetic outflow, induce pathological changes in the arterial walls, and increase cerebral metabolism as well as oxygen consumption.

Further Reading: Ohba S, Nakagawa T, Murakami H. Concurrent Graves' disease and intracranial arterial stenosis/occlusion: special considerations regarding the state of thyroid function, etiology, and treatment. *Neurosurg Rev.* 2011;34(3):297–304

47.

C Abducens n

The patient has sagittal sinus thrombosis with increased venous congestion and increased ICP. The most common cranial neuropathy with increased ICP is the abducens (VI) nerve.

48.

A PCOM aneurysm

Partially thrombosed aneurysms can often appear as hyperdense masses adjacent to or within the sellar region. PCOM aneurysm (*arrow*) can also present with IIIrd nerve palsy causing mydriasis. Vascular imaging is warranted with CTA, MRA, or DSA.

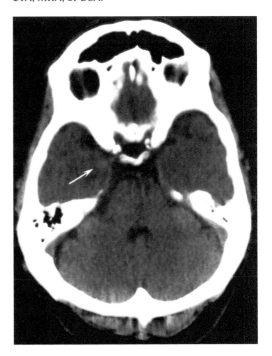

49.

A Verocay bodies

Schwannomas are benign nerve sheath tumors usually presenting with pain. MRI reveals an intradural extramedullary enhancing lesion. Histologically they demonstrate a higher cellular Antoni A pattern with palisading nuclei around Verocay bodies with areas of less cellular Antoni B pattern with looser stroma and myxoid changes. Rosenthal fibers are seen in pilocytic astrocytoma, mitosis and necrosis in malignant tumors, cuboidal cells on myxoid cores in myxopapillary ependymomas, and dilated vessels with thin walls in hemangioblastoma.

50.

E Atretic cephalocele

Atretic cephaloceles are small subcutaneous scalp lesions that consist of dura, fibrous tissue, and dysplastic brain tissue presenting in infants and young children. They are palpable midline soft tissue masses thought to represent involution of a true cephalocele connected to the dura mater via a fibrous stalk. Radiographically there is a CSF tract and vertical falcine vein pointing toward the subcutaneous scalp mass. Sinus pericranii is a venous extracranial lesion that communicates with a dural sinus and gets smaller with erect posture (unless thrombosed). Eosinophilic granuloma (Langerhans cell histiocytosis) present as lytic skull lesions in children, with more involvement of the inner table (beveled edges). Epidermoid cysts have sclerotic margins on X-ray and restricted diffusion on MRI.

51.

C One plexiform neurofibroma

The clinical diagnosis of NF-1 is made if two or more of the following criteria are present: six or more café-au-lait spots, axillary or inguinal freckling, two or more neurofibromas or one plexiform neurofibroma, optic nerve glioma (seen on MRI), two or more iris hamartomas (Lisch nodules), sphenoid dysplasia or long bone abnormalities, and a first-degree relative with NF-1.

52.

E 5

There are five primary ossification centers of the axis: two in the vertebral arch, one in the vertebral body, and two along the dens.

53.

A The patient has a respiratory acidosis.

The patient has a pH of 7.18 and $PaCO_2$ of 68 mmHg, so respiratory acidosis. Since HCO_3 is normal (24 mEq/L), there is no metabolic compensation.

54.

E 142 mEq/L

The patient has diabetic ketoacidosis. The classic correction formula is: corrected sodium = measured sodium + [1.6 (glucose − 100) / 100]. Corrected Na = 126 + [1.6 (1100 − 100) / 100] = 142 mEq/L.

55.

B Potassium channels remain open.

Voltage-gated potassium channels open to terminate the action potential by repolarizing the membrane with potassium ions moving out of the cell, while sodium channels are closed. During the absolute refractory period, no stimulus can generate an action potential, while during the relative refractory period, a supra normal stimulus can. Local anesthetics block sodium channels and prevent an action potential (**Fig. 27**).

56.

E An action potential can only be initiated once the resting potential reaches −25 mV.

The resting membrane potential is typically −90 mV for the axon and −65 mV at the axon hillock and cell body. An action potential threshold is typically around −65 mV for the axon, −45 mV at the axon hillock, and −35 mV at the cell body. The axon hillock has the highest concentration of sodium channels and is the most excitable part of the neuron.

57.

D Layer V

Layer V, the internal pyramidal layer, contains large Betz cells whose axons travel to the internal capsule, brain stem, and spinal cord. Fibers emanating from the motor cortex form the corticospinal and corticobulbar tracts. Layer VI sends efferents to the thalamus while layer IV is the main afferent input. Layer III connects to commissural fibers (corpus callosum) while layers I–III contain intrahemispheric association fibers (**Fig. 3**).

58.

D Glycine

Descending glycinergic and GABAergic systems contribute to inhibition of nociceptive signaling especially in the dorsal horn of the spinal cord. The role of serotonin can be variable depending on the receptors.

Further Reading: Ossipov MH, Dussor GO, Porreca F. Central modulation of pain. *J Clin Invest.* 2010 Nov;120(11):3779–3787

Ossipov MH, Morimura K, Porreca F. Descending pain modulation and chronification of pain. *Curr Opin Support Palliat Care* 2014 Jun;8(2):143–151

59.

A Lamina I (marginal nucleus)

Fast (sharp) Aδ pain fibers enter into lamina I and utilize glutamate as neurotransmitter while slow (burning) C pain fibers enter into lamina II and utilize substance P (**Fig. 15**).

60.

C Increased urine coproporphyrin III

Coproporphyria with increased levels of coproporphyrin III occurs in the urine in clinical lead (Pb) poisoning and with exposure to Pb even without clinically apparent symptoms and is most diagnostic and consistent with Pb poisoning. Other findings include increased urinary delta-aminolevulinic acid, increased blood lead level (BLL), and basophilic stippling of RBCs (**Table 30**). Anemia of Pb toxicity is either normocytic or microcytic. Megaloblastic anemia occurs in B12 and folate deficiency as well as Dilantin toxicity (**Table 34**). TIBC is increased in iron-deficiency anemia.

Section II.   Diagrams

Lateral Surface

Medial Surface

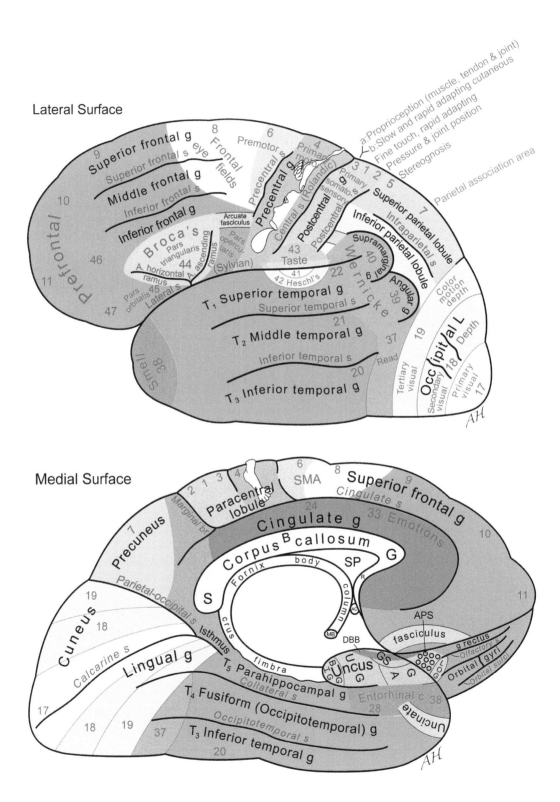

Fig. 1 Cerebral cortex, lateral aspect. Anterior; g, gyrus; L, lobe; s, sulcus; The arcuate fasciculus connects Broca's area to Wernicke's area. The numbers correspond to the Brodmann's areas. Copyright Amgad Hanna.

Fig. 2 Cerebral cortex, medial, and inferior aspect. AC, anterior commissure; APS, anterior perforated substance; B, body; BG, band of Giacomini; br, branch; c, cortex; DBB, diagonal band of Broca; G, genu; g, gyrus; GA, gyrus ambiens; GS, gyrus semilunaris; IG, intralimbic gyrus; LOG, lateral olfactory gyrus; MB, mammillary body; R, rostrum; s, sulcus; S, splenium; SMA, supplementary motor area; UG, uncinated gyrus. The amygdala is deep to GA, GS, and UG. The prepiriform region includes LOG, GA, GS, UG, BG, and IG. The prepiriform lobe includes the prepiriform region plus the entorhinal cortex. The uncinate fasciculus connects the orbitofrontal cortex to the temporal pole. The numbers correspond to the Brodmann's areas. Copyright Amgad Hanna. Published with permission.

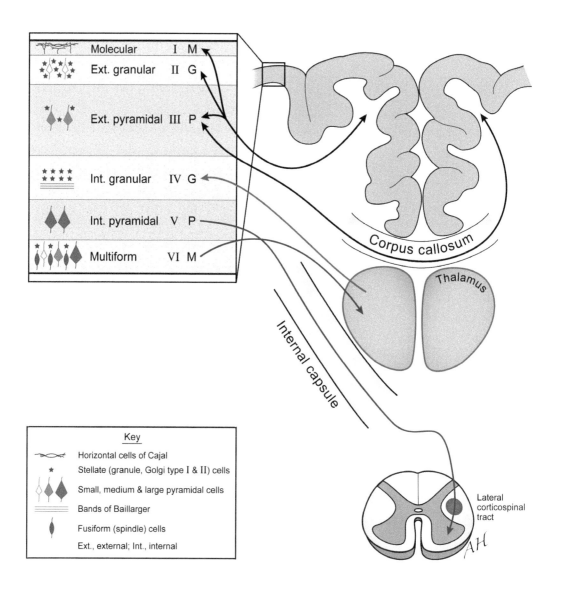

Molecular	I	M
Ext. granular	II	G
Ext. pyramidal	III	P
Int. granular	IV	G
Int. pyramidal	V	P
Multiform	VI	M

Corpus callosum

Thalamus

Internal capsule

Lateral corticospinal tract

Key

Horizontal cells of Cajal

Stellate (granule, Golgi type I & II) cells

Small, medium & large pyramidal cells

Bands of Baillarger

Fusiform (spindle) cells

Ext., external; Int., internal

Fig. 3 Cerebral cortex layers (Lorente de Nó). Layers I–III are involved in ipsilateral cortical connections. Layer III is involved in contralateral cortical connections (commissural). Layer IV is the major afferent pathway. Layer V is the major efferent pathway to the brain stem and spinal cord. Layer VI is the efferent pathway to the thalamus. Copyright Amgad Hanna.

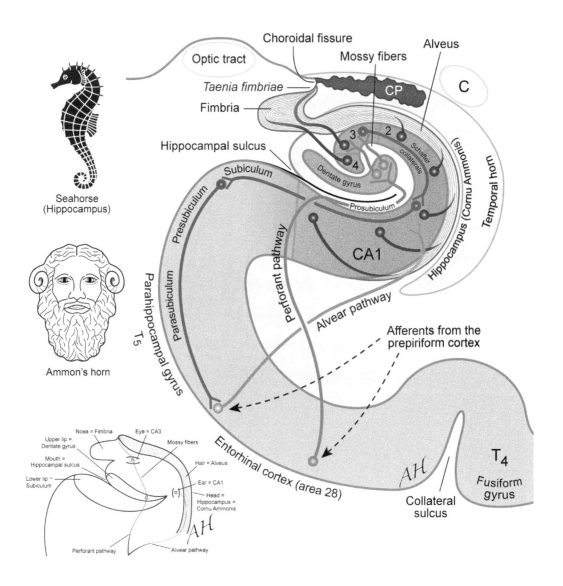

Choroidal fissure

Optic tract

Mossy fibers

Alveus

Taenia fimbriae

CP

C

Fimbria

Hippocampal sulcus

3 2

Schafer collaterals

Subiculum

Dentate gyrus

Prosubiculum

Presubiculum

4

Hippocampus (Cornu Ammonis)

Temporal horn

Seahorse (Hippocampus)

Parasubiculum

Perforant pathway

CA1

Parahippocampal gyrus

T5

Alvear pathway

Ammon's horn

Afferents from the prepiriform cortex

Nose = Fimbria

Eye = CA3

Upper lip = Dentate gyrus

Mossy fibers

Mouth = Hippocampal sulcus

Hair = Alveus

Lower lip = Subiculum

Ear = CA1

Head = Hippocampus = Cornu Ammonis

Entorhinal cortex (area 28)

AH

T4

Fusiform gyrus

Perforant pathway

Alvear pathway

AH

Collateral sulcus

Fig. 4 **Hippocampus.** The hippocampus is likened to the seahorse and Ammon's horn (Cornu Ammonis, CA). Also, the hippocampus and its pathways are likened to a human face (bottom left). C, caudate; CP, choroid plexus. Copyright Amgad Hanna.

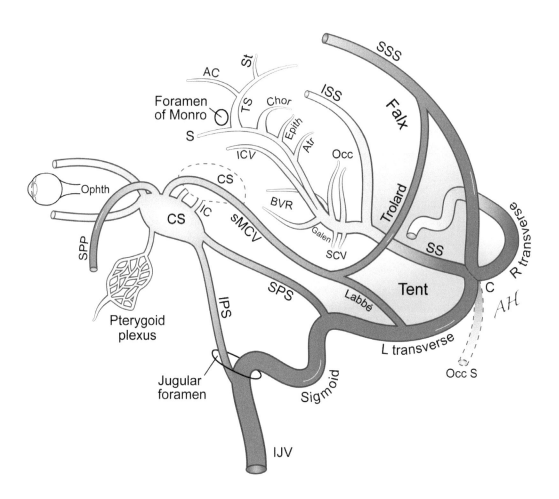

Fig. 5 Major intracranial veins and their connections. AC, anterior caudate v; Atr, atrial v; BVR, basal v of Rosenthal; C, venous confluence (corresponds to the torcular Herophili on the skull); Chor, choroidal v; CS, cavernous sinus; Epith, epithalamic v; IC, intercavernous (coronary) sinuses; ICV, internal cerebral v; IJV, internal jugular v; IPS, inferior petrosal sinus; ISS, inferior sagittal sinus; Occ, occipital vv; Occ S, occipital sinus; Ophth, ophthalmic vv; S, septal v; SCV, superior cerebellar vv; sMCV, superficial middle cerebral v; SPP, sphenoparietal sinus of Breschet; SPS, superior petrosal sinus; SS, straight sinus; SSS, superior sagittal sinus; St, striatal v; Tent, tentorium cerebelli; TS, thalamostriate v. The septal v meets the thalamostriate v at the foramen of Monro. In the right lateral ventricle, the thalamostriate v is to the right of the choroid plexus. At the venous confluence, the superior sagittal sinus and straight sinus may both drain into both transverse sinuses or the superior sagittal sinus drains to the right transverse sinus and the straight sinus to the left. Copyright Amgad Hanna.

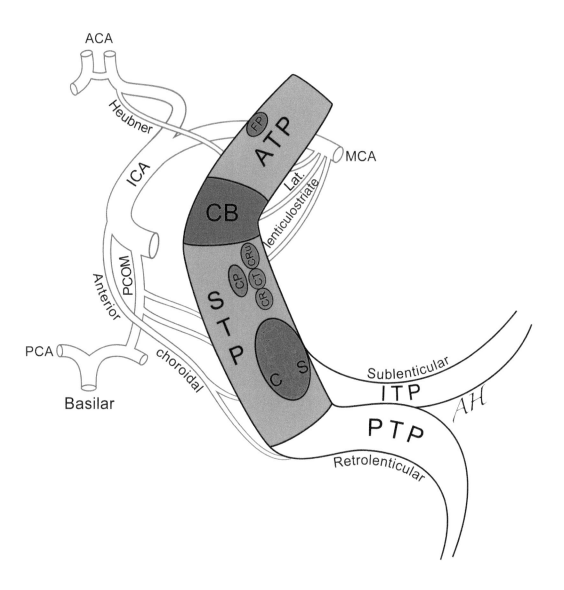

Fig. 6 Internal capsule and its blood supply. ACA, anterior cerebral artery; ATP, anterior thalamic peduncle; CB, corticobulbar tract, occupies the genu; CP, corticopontine fibers; CR, corticorubral tract; Cru, corticoreticular; CS, corticospinal tract, occupies the posterior half of the posterior limb, somatotopically organized with the legs posteriorly; CT, corticotectal tract; FP, frontopontine fibers; ICA, internal carotid artery; ITP, inferior thalamic peduncle, auditory projections; Lat., lateral; MCA, middle cerebral artery; PCA, posterior cerebral artery; PCOM, posterior communicating artery; PTP, posterior thalamic peduncle, visual projections; STP, superior thalamic peduncle, carries general somatic sensation. Copyright Amgad Hanna.

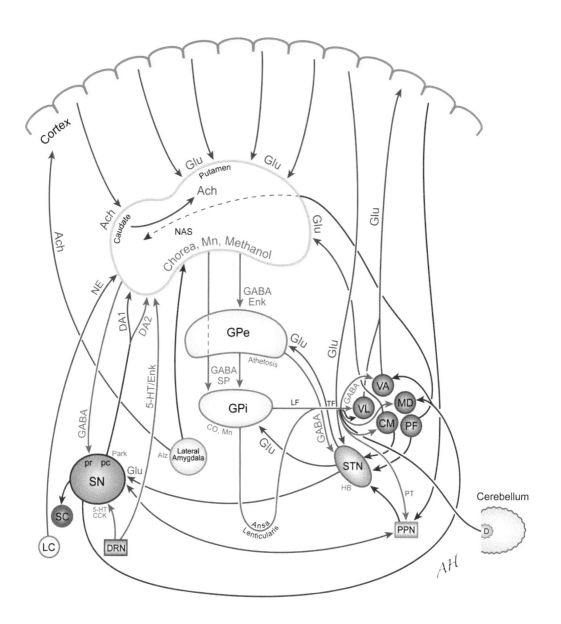

Fig. 7 Basal ganglia and their connections. 5-HT, serotonin (5-hydroxytryptamine); Ach, acetylcholine; CCK, cholecystokinin; Alz, Alzheimer's disease; CM, centromedian thalamic nucleus; CO, carbon monoxide poisoning; D, dentate nucleus; DA, dopamine; DRN, dorsal raphe nucleus; Enk, enkephalins; GABA, γ-aminobutyric acid; Glu, glutamate; GPe, globus pallidus externus; GPi, globus pallidus internus; HB, hemiballismus; LC, locus ceruleus; LF, lenticular fasciculus (Forel's Field H2, FFH2); MD, medial dorsal thalamic nucleus; Mn, manganese toxicity; NAS, nucleus accumbens septi; NE, norepinephrine; Park, Parkinson's disease; PF, parafascicular thalamic nucleus; PPN, pedunculopontine nucleus; PT, pallidotegmental fibers; SC, superior colliculus; SN, substantia nigra: pc, pars compacta and pr, pars reticulata; SP, substance P; STN, subthalamic nucleus; TF, thalamic fasciculus (FFH1); VA, ventral anterior thalamic nucleus; VL, ventral lateral thalamic nucleus. *Arrow colors:* blue, excitatory; red, inhibitory. Archistriatum, amygdala; paleostriatum, globus pallidus; neostriatum, caudate and putamen. The caudate, putamen and amygdala are parts of the telencephalon, while the GP and STN are parts of the diencephalon. Copyright Amgad Hanna.

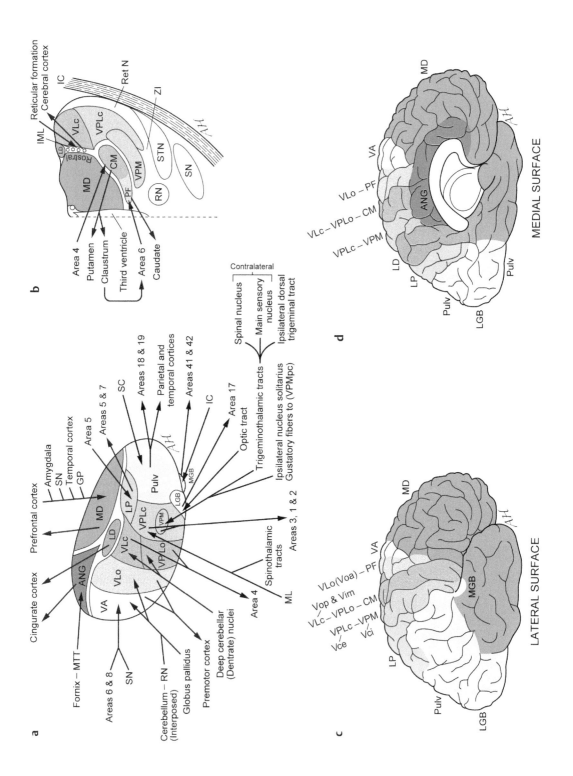

Fig. 8 Major thalamic nuclei and their projections. ANG, anterior nuclear group; CM, centromedian; GP, globus pallidus; IC, internal capsule; IML, internal medullary lamina; LD, lateral dorsal; LGB, lateral geniculate body; LP, lateral posterior; MD, medial dorsal; MGB, medial geniculate body; ML, medial lemniscus; MTT, mammil-lothalamic tract; PF, parafascicular; Pulv, pulvinar; Ret N, reticular nucleus; RN, red nucleus; SC, superior colliculus; SN, substantia nigra; STN, subthalamic nucleus; VA, ventral anterior; VLc, ventral lateral, pars caudalis (= Vop, ventralis oralis posterior and Vim, ventralis intermediate); VLo, ventral lateral, pars oralis (= Voa, ventralis ora-lis anterior); VPLc, ventral posterolateral, pars caudalis (= Vce, ventralis caudalis externus); VPLo, ventral posterolateral, pars oralis; VPM, ventral posteromedial (= Vci, ventralis caudalis internus); ZI, zona incerta. The intralaminar nuclei include CM which connects area 4 to putamen, PF which connects area 6 to caudate, and rostral nuclei which connect the reticular formation to the cerebral cortex and play a role in the awake state. Copyright Amgad Hanna.

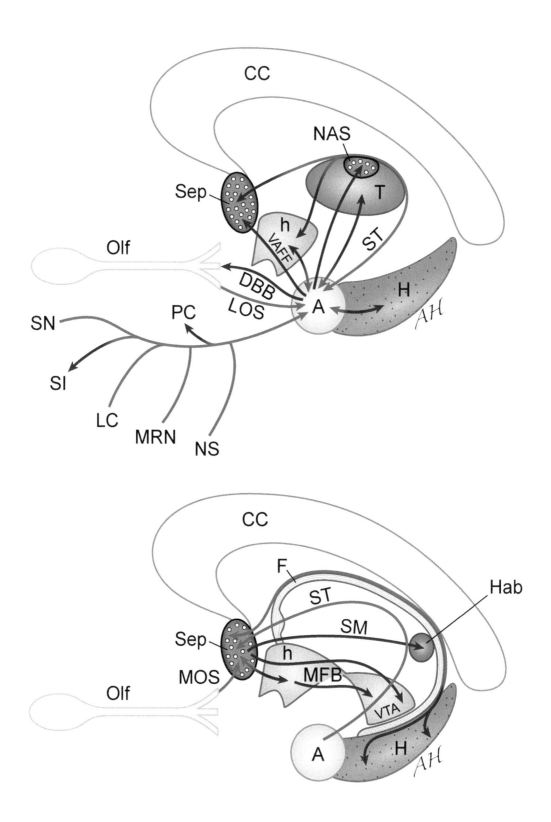

Fig. 9 Amygdala (top) and septal nuclei (bottom) connections. Arrow colors: blue, efferents; red, afferents. A, amygdala; CC, corpus callosum; DBB, diagonal band of Broca; F, fornix; h, hypothalamus; H, hippocampus; Hab, habenula; LC, locus ceruleus; LOS, lateral olfactory stria; MFB, medial forebrain bundle; MOS, medial olfactory stria; MRN, median raphe nucleus; NAS, nucleus accumbens septi; NS, nucleus solitarius; Olf, olfactory tract; PC, pan-cortex; Sep, septal nuclei; SI, substantia innominata; SM, stria medullaris; SN, substantia nigra; ST, stria terminalis; T, thalamus; VAFF, ventral amygdalofugal fibers; VTA, ventral tegmental area. Copyright Amgad Hanna.

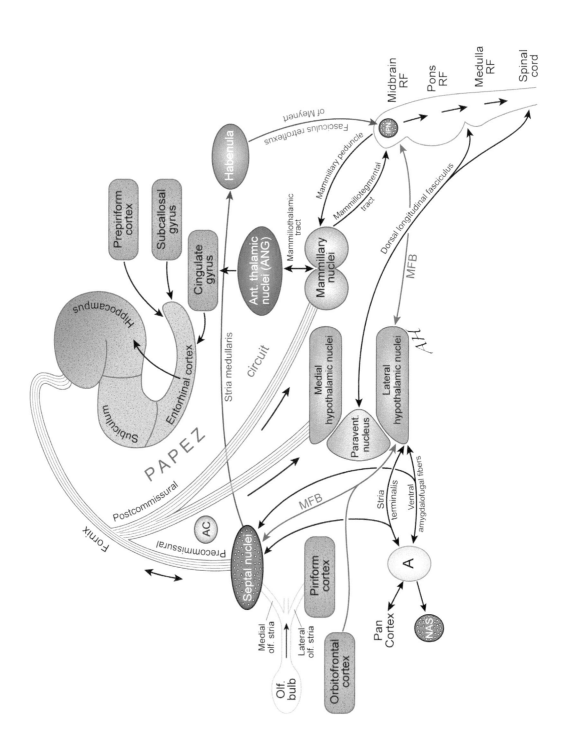

Fig. 10 Limbic system and its connections. A, amygdala; AC, anterior commissure; ANG, anterior nuclear group (thalamus); IPN, interpeduncular nuclei; MFB, medial forebrain bundle; NAS, nucleus accumbens septi; Olf, olfactory; Paravent, paraventricular; RF, reticular formation. Copyright Amgad Hanna.

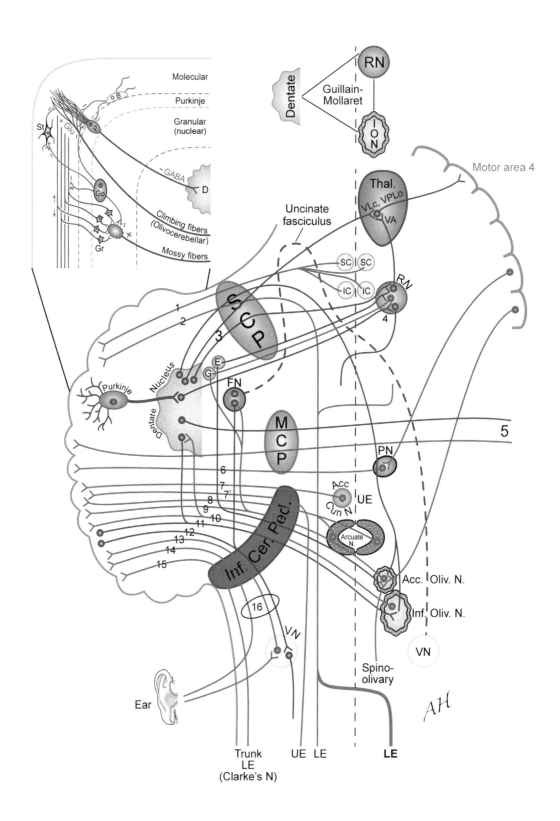

Fig. 11 Cerebellar tracts. 1, tectocerebellar tract; 2, ventral spinocerebellar tract (mostly crossed); 3, dentatothalamic tract; 4, dentatorubrospinal tract. 1-4 pass through the superior cerebellar peduncle (SCP, brachium conjunctivum). 5, cerebellopontocerebellar tract; 6, corticopontocerebellar tract. 5 and 6 pass through the middle cerebellar peduncle (MCP). 7, posterior (dorsal) external arcuate fibers, this is the cuneocerebellar tract arising from the accessory cuneate nucleus (Acc Cun N), 7′, rostral spinocerebellar tract; 8, anterior (ventral) external arcuate fibers; 9, parolivocerebellar tract, arises from the accessory olivary nucleus (Acc. Oliv. N.); 10, olivocerebellar tract (climbing fibers), arises from the inferior olivary nucleus (Inf. Oliv. N.); 11, cerebello-olivary tract; 12, cerebellovestibular (fastigiobulbar) tract; 13, indirect vestibulocerebellar tract; 14, direct vestibulocerebellar tract; 15, dorsal spinocerebellar tract; 16, juxtarestiform body. 7–16 pass through the inferior cerebellar peduncle (Inf. Cer. Ped.) or restiform body. B, basket cells; D, dentate nucleus; E, emboliform nucleus; FN, fastigial nucleus; G, globose nucleus; Glu, glutamate; Go, Golgi cells; Gr, granule cells; IC, inferior colliculus; ION, inferior olivary nucleus; LE, lower extremity; N, nucleus; P, Purkinje cells; PN, pontine nuclei; RN, red nucleus; SC; superior colliculus; St, stellate cells; Thal., thalamus: (VA, ventral anterior nucleus; VLc, ventral lateral nucleus, pars caudalis; VPLo, ventral posterolateral nucleus, pars oralis); UE, upper extremity; VN, vestibular nuclei. Note that granule cells, climbing fibers and mossy fibers are excitatory. Disruption of the Guillain–Mollaret triangle causes oculopalatal myoclonus. Copyright Amgad Hanna.

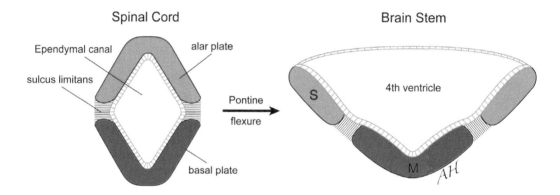

Spinal Cord   Brain Stem

Ependymal canal   alar plate

sulcus limitans

Pontine
flexure

basal plate

4th ventricle

S

M   *AH*

Fig. 12 Pontine flexure. Pontine flexure causes lateral walls of the medulla and pons to move outwards like an open book. From the basal plate develops the efferent (motor, M) system and from the alar plate develops the afferent (sensory, S) system. The two plates are separated by the sulcus limitans. Copyright Amgad Hanna.

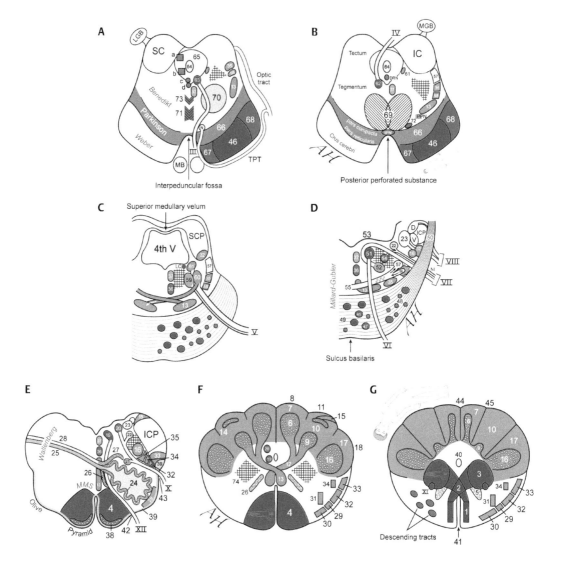

Fig. 13 Brain stem axial cuts. A. Midbrain, superior colliculus (SC) level. **B.** Midbrain, inferior colliculus (IC) level. **C.** Upper pons. **D.** Lower pons. **E.** Open medulla oblongata. **F.** Closed medulla oblongata, sensory decussation. **G.** Closed medulla oblongata, motor decussation. 1, ventral corticospinal tract; 2, pyramidal decussation (75%); 3, lateral corticospinal tract; 4, pyramid; 5, detached anterior horn (supraspinal nucleus); 6, gracile nucleus; 7, gracile fasciculus; 8, gracile tubercle; 9, cuneate nucleus; 10, cuneate fasciculus; 11, cuneate tubercle; 12, internal arcuate fibers; 13, medial lemniscus; 14, accessory cuneate nucleus; 15, posterior external arcuate fibers (cuneocerebellar tract); 16, spinal nucleus of V; 17, spinal tract of V; 18, tuber cinereum; 19, XII nucleus; 20, dorsal nucleus of X; 21, nucleus ambiguus; 22, nucleus solitarius; 23, vestibular nuclei; D and V, dorsal and ventral cochlear nuclei; 24, inferior olivary nucleus; 25, olivocerebellar tract (climbing fibers); 26 and 27, medial and dorsal accessory olivary nuclei; 28, parolivocerebellar tract; 29, spino-olivary tract; 30 and 31, ventral and lateral spinothalamic tracts; 32 and 33, ventral and dorsal spinocerebellar tracts; 34, spinotectal tract; 35, spinal lemniscus; 36, tectospinal tract; 37, medial longitudinal fasciculus (MLF); 38, arcuate nucleus; 39, anterior external arcuate fibers; 40, central canal (CSF); 41, anterior median fissure; 42, anterolateral sulcus; 43, posterolateral sulcus; 44, posterior median sulcus; 45, posterior intermediate sulcus; 46, pyramidal tract (corticobulbar and corticospinal), legs are lateral, 47, corticopontine fibers; 48, pontine nuclei; 49, transverse pontine fibers; 50, middle cerebellar peduncle; 51, VI nucleus; 52, motor nucleus of VII; 53, facial colliculus; 54, superior salivary nucleus; 55, trapezoid body and nuclei; 56, superior olivary nucleus; 57, lateral lemniscus; 58, trigeminal lemniscus (crossed); 59, motor nucleus of V; 60, main sensory nucleus of V; 61, mesencephalic nucleus of V; 62, nucleus of IV; 63, nucleus of III; 64, cerebral aqueduct of Sylvius; 65, periaqueductal gray matter; 66, substantia nigra; 67, frontopontine fibers; 68, temporo-, parieto-, and occipito-pontine fibers; 69, decussation of the superior cerebellar peduncle (SCP) of Wernekinck; 70, red nucleus; 71, rubrospinal decussation; 72, rubrospinal tract; 73, tectospinal decussation; 74, reticular formation; a, nucleus of posterior commissure; b, Darkschewitsch nucleus; c, Interstitial nucleus of Cajal; d, RiMLF (rostral interstitial nucleus of MLF); 4th V, fourth ventricle; DRN, dorsal raphe nucleus (5-HT, CCK, Enk); IPN, interpeduncular nucleus; LC, locus ceruleus (NE); LGB, lateral geniculate body; MB, mammillary bodies; MGB, medial geniculate body; NI, nervus intermedius; PPN, pedunculopontine nucleus (Ach); TPT, tractus peduncularis transversus (N, nucleus of TPT). Brain stem stroke syndromes: Benedikt: red nucleus (contralateral ataxia) and III n. (Of note, Claude's syndrome also involves the red nucleus and III n.) Weber: pyramidal tract (crossed hemiplegia) and III n. Millard–Gubler: crossed hemiplegia and VI and VII palsy. MMS: medial medullary syndrome (Dejerine): crossed hemiplegia, medial lemniscus (contralateral loss of touch and proprioception), XII n. Lateral medullary syndrome (Wallenberg): spinal lemniscus (contralateral loss of pain and temperature sensation) and ipsilateral: ataxia, Horner's, IX, X, XI, V (decreased taste, gag, hoarseness, dysphagia, loss of pain, and temperature of the face). Copyright Amgad Hanna.

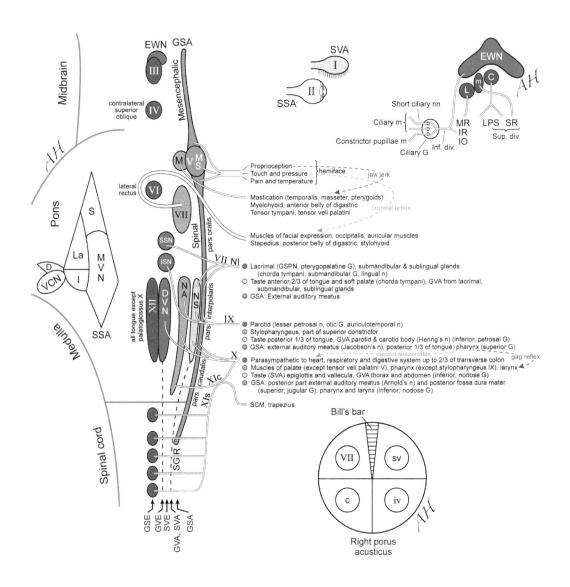

Fig. 14 Cranial nn. GSA, general somatic afferents (pain, temperature, touch, pressure, proprioception: V, VII, IX, and X); GSE, general somatic efferents (motor to skeletal muscles III, IV, VI, and XII); GVA, general visceral afferents (nucleus solitarius [NS], parasympathetic afferents); GVE, general visceral efferents (parasympathetics, III, VII [superior salivary nucleus, SSN to chorda tympani], IX [inferior salivary nucleus, ISN] and X [dorsal vagal nucleus, DVN]); SSA, special somatic afferents (vision II and hearing VIII); SVA, special visceral afferents (smell I and taste [nucleus solitarius]: VII, IX, and X); SVE, special visceral efferents (motor to branchial arch muscles V, VII, and nucleus ambiguus [NA]: IX, X, and XI). Oculomotor n components include Edinger–Westphal nucleus (EWN, parasympathetic), central nucleus (C) to levator palpebrae superioris (LPS) bilaterally, medial nucleus (m) to contralateral superior rectus (SR), and lateral nucleus (L) to ipsilateral medial rectus (MR), inferior rectus (IR), and inferior oblique (IO). In the porus acusticus (internal auditory meatus), VII is cranial to cochlear (c) (7up, Coke down) and medial to superior vestibular (sv); the latter is separated from VII by the Bill's bar. Inferior vestibular (iv) is caudal to sv. D, dorsal cochlear nucleus; G, ganglion; GSPN, greater superficial petrosal n; I, inferior vestibular nucleus; Inf. div., inferior division; La, lateral vestibular nucleus; MS, main sensory nucleus of V (touch and pressure); MVN, medial vestibular nucleus; NI, nervus intermedius; S, superior vestibular nucleus; SCM, sternocleidomastoid; SGR, substantia gelatinosa of Rolando; Sup. div., superior division; VCN, ventral cochlear nucleus. Copyright Amgad Hanna.

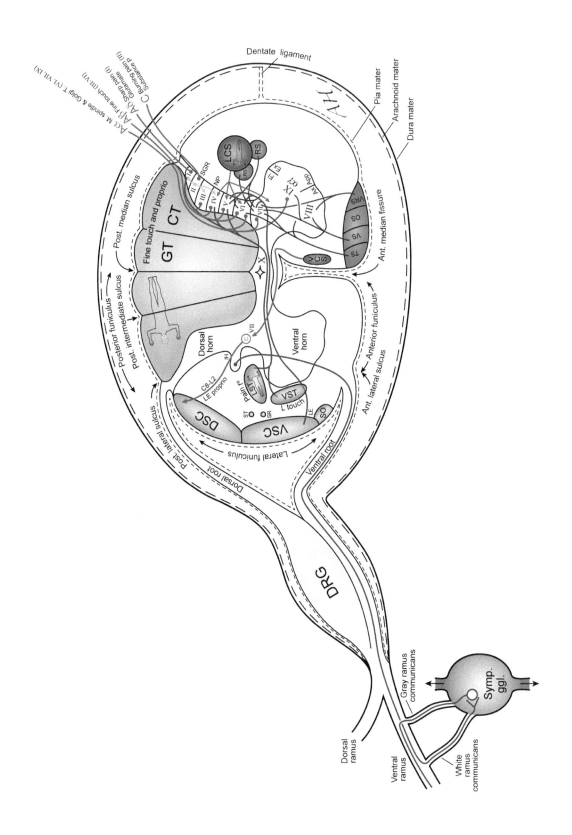

Fig. 15 Spinal cord. Ant., anterior; Ax, axial muscles (medial); App, appendicular muscles (lateral); C, Clarke's nucleus; CT, cuneate tract; DRG, dorsal root ganglion (sensory); DSC, dorsal spinocerebellar; Ex, extensors (ventral); Fl, flexors (dorsal); Golgi T., Golgi tendon organ; GT, gracile tract; IH, intermediate horn; LCS, lateral corticospinal tract (legs lateral); LE proprio, lower extremity proprioception; LRS, lateral reticulospinal tract; LST, lateral spinothalamic tract (pain and temperature [t°]), legs lateral; M. spindle, muscle spindle; NP, nucleus proprius, layers III and IV; OS, olivospinal; Post., posterior; RS, rubrospinal tract; SGR, substantia gelatinosa of Rolando (Substance P), layer II; SO, spino-olivary; SR, spinoreticular; ST, spinotectal; Symp. ggl., sympathetic ganglion; TS, tectospinal; VCS, ventral corticospinal; VRS, ventral reticulospinal; VS, vestibulospinal; VSC, ventral spinocerebellar; VST, ventral spinothalamic tract (light [L] touch); I–X, Rexed laminae. Copyright Amgad Hanna.

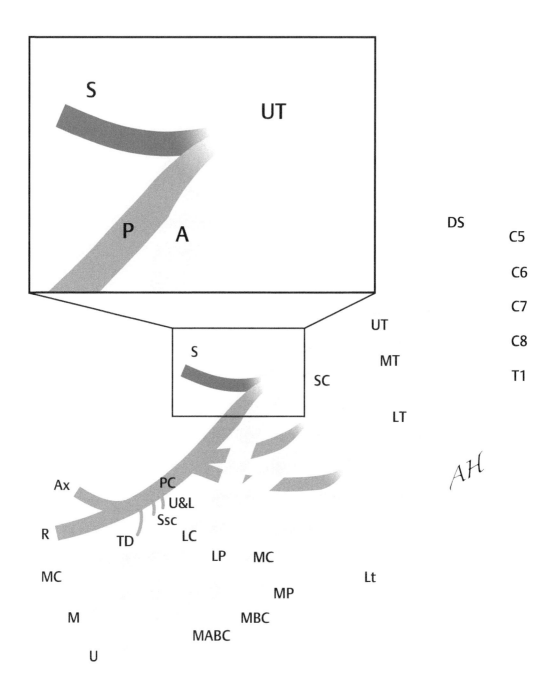

S

UT

P   A

DS

C5

C6

C7

C8

T1

UT

S

MT

SC

LT

AH

Ax   PC

U&L

Ssc

R   TD   LC

LP   MC   Lt

MC

MP

M   MBC

MABC

U

Fig. 16 Brachial plexus. New diagram of the brachial plexus, taking into account the SPA arrangement of the trifurcation of the upper trunk. DS, dorsal scapular n; Lt, long thoracic n; UT, upper trunk; MT, middle trunk; LT, lower trunk; SC, n to subclavius; S, suprascapular n; P, posterior division of upper trunk; A, anterior division of upper trunk; PC, posterior cord; LC, lateral cord; MC, medial cord; U&L Ssc, upper and lower subscapular nn; TD, thoracodorsal n; Ax, axillary n; R, radial n; LP, lateral pectoral n; MC, musculo-cutaneous n; M, median n; U, ulnar n; MP, medial pectoral n; MBC, medial brachial cutaneous n; MABC, medial antebrachial cutaneous n. Copyright Amgad Hanna, reproduced from: The SPA arrangement of the branches of the upper trunk of the brachial plexus: a correction of a longstanding misconception and a new diagram of the brachial plexus. Hanna A. *J Neurosurg* 2016 Aug;125(2):350–354. Published with permission.

Disclaimer: Until everybody is familiar with this diagram, unfortunately the older diagrams may still show on tests. Previous diagrams misrepresent the branching pattern of the upper trunk as suprascapular, anterior division then posterior division from cranial to caudal, which is anatomically incorrect.

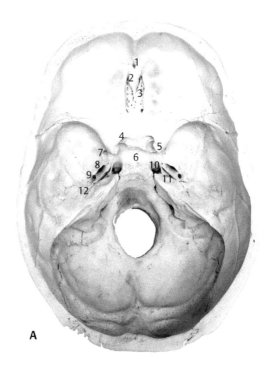

A

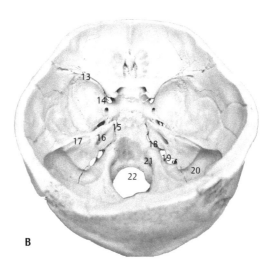

B

Fig. 17 Interior view of the bony skull base. A. 1, foramen cecum; 2, crista galli; 3, cribriform plate of ethmoid (for cranial n I); 4, optic canal (II, ophthalmic a); 5, anterior clinoid process; 6, sella turcica (hypophyseal fossa); 7, foramen rotundum (maxillary division of V [V_2], a of foramen rotundum); 8, foramen ovale (mandibular division of V [V_3], lesser petrosal n [IX], accessory meningeal a); 9, foramen spinosum (middle meningeal a, meningeal branch of V_3); 10, foramen lacerum (covered with cartilage on top of which lies the ICA; 11, Meckel's cave (trigeminal [Gasserian] ganglion); 12, groove for GSPN (greater superficial petrosal n of VII). **B.** 13, groove for sphenoparietal sinus; 14, superior orbital fissure (outside annulus of Zinn: LFT; Lacrimal and Frontal branches of the ophthalmic division of V, Trochlear n + superior ophthalmic v. Inside the annulus of Zinn: nasociliary branch of V, superior and inferior divisions of III, VI); 15, Dorello's canal (VI); 16, internal acoustic meatus (VII, VIII, nervus intermedius, internal auditory [labyrinthine] a, and rarely a persistent otic a); 17, groove for superior petrosal sinus (between cavernous sinus and sigmoid); 18, groove for inferior petrosal sinus (between cavernous sinus and IJV); 19, jugular foramen (inferior petrosal sinus, IX, X, XI, IJV, occasionally posterior meningeal a); 20, groove for sigmoid sinus; 21, hypoglossal canal (XII, occasionally posterior meningeal a, and rarely a persistent hypoglossal a); 22, foramen magnum (cervicomedullary junction with meningeal coverings, vertebral aa [x2], anterior spinal a, posterior spinal aa [x2], spinal root of accessory n [x2], craniocervical ligaments [tectorial membrane, cruciate ligament superior extension], occasionally posterior meningeal a).

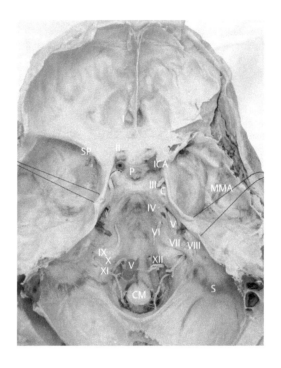

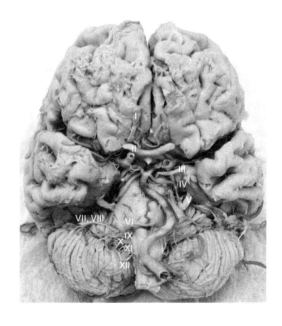

Fig. 18 Interior view of the skull base showing cranial nerves. I, olfactory n; II, optic n; III, oculomotor n; IV, trochlear n; V, trigeminal n; VI, abducens n; VII, facial n; VIII, vestibulocochlear n; IX, glossopharyngeal n; X, vagus n; XI, accessory n; XII, hypoglossal n; C, cavernous sinus; CM, cervicomedullary junction; ICA, internal carotid a; MMA, middle meningeal a; P, pituitary stalk; S, sigmoid sinus; SP, sphenoparietal sinus; V, vertebral a.

Fig. 19 Cranial nerves on the undersurface of the brain. I, olfactory n; II, optic n; III, oculomotor n; IV, trochlear n; V, trigeminal n; VI, abducens n; VII, facial n; VIII, vestibulocochlear n; IX, glossopharyngeal n; X, vagus n; XI, accessory n; XII, hypoglossal n.

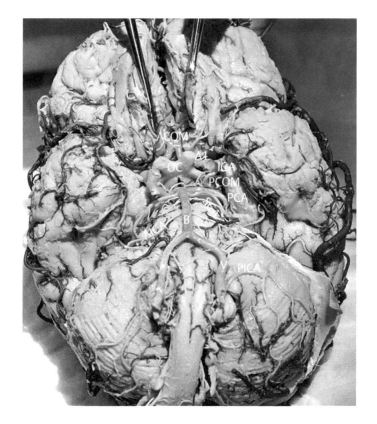

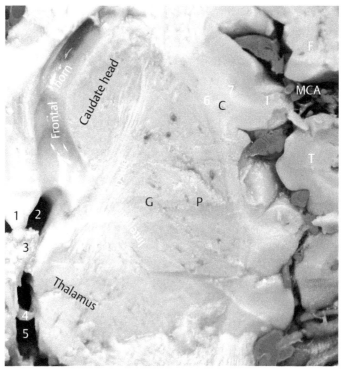

Fig. 20 Circle of Willis. A1, anterior cerebral a, first segment; ACOM, anterior communicating a; AICA, anterior inferior cerebellar a; B, basilar a; ICA, internal carotid a; OC, optic chiasm; PCA, posterior cerebral a; PCOM, posterior communicating a; PICA, posterior inferior cerebellar a; SCA, superior cerebellar a; V, vertebral a.

Fig. 21 Axial cut through the basal ganglia. 1, Fornix; 2, foramen of Monro; 3, choroid plexus; 4, interthalamic adhesion; 5, third ventricle; 6, external capsule; 7, extreme capsule; C, claustrum; F; frontal lobe; G, globus pallidus; I, insula; MCA, middle cerebral a; P, putamen; T, temporal lobe.

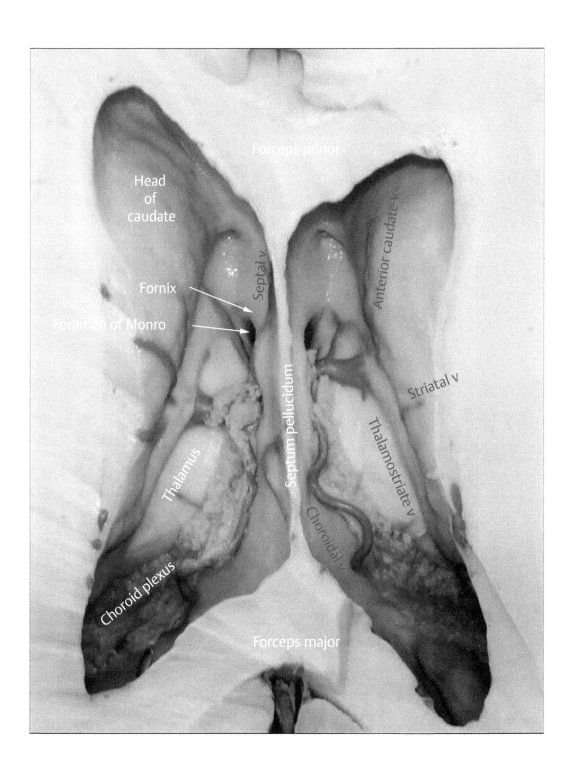

Fig. 22 Superior view of the floor of the lateral ventricles. Note that in the *right* lateral ventricle, the thalamostriate v is to the *right* of the choroid plexus. Also note that the fornix forms the superior and anterior boundary of the foramen of Monro.

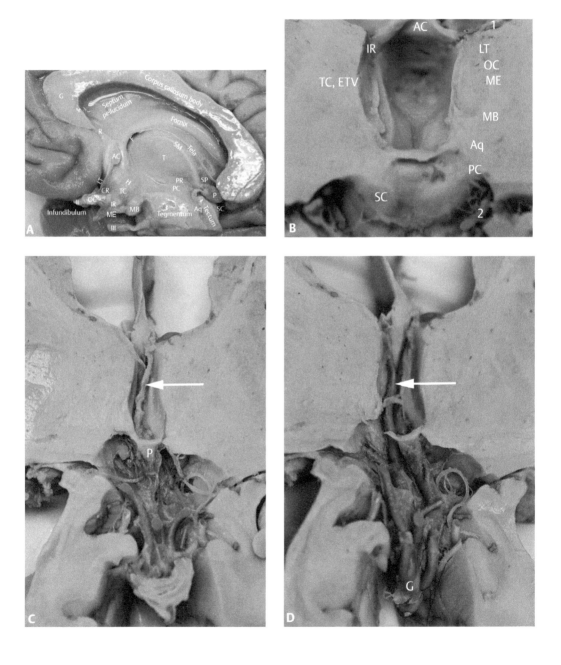

Fig. 23 Third ventricle. A. Sagittal view. **B.** The floor and anterior wall of the third ventricle. 1, Thalamostriate v; 2, basal v of Rosenthal; AC, anterior commissure; Aq, cerebral aqueduct of Sylvius; CR, chiasmatic (supraoptic) recess; F, interventricular foramen of Monro; G, genu; H, hypothalamus; IR, infundibular recess; LT, lamina terminalis; MB, mammillary body; ME, median eminence; OC, optic chiasm; P, pineal gland; PC, posterior commissure; PR, pineal recess; R, rostrum; S, splenium; SC, superior colliculus; SM, stria medullaris thalami; SP, suprapineal recess; T, thalamus; TC, tuber cinereum which is the site for endoscopic third ventriculostomy (ETV) between *MB* and *ME*; Tela, tela choroidea in the roof of the third ventricle. **C.** Choroid plexus (*arrow*) in the roof of the third ventricle. **D.** Internal cerebral veins (*arrow*) in the roof of the third ventricle. G, v of Galen.

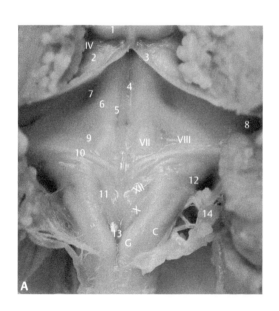

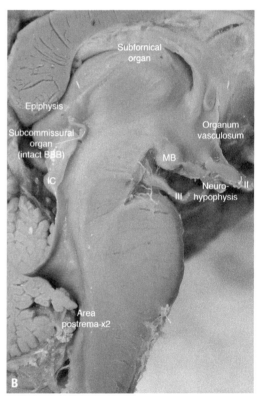

Fig. 24 A. Fourth ventricle floor. Note the rhomboid shape. 1, Inferior colliculus; 2, superior cerebellar peduncle; 3, superior medullary velum; 4, median sulcus; 5, medial eminence; 6, sulcus limitans; 7, locus ceruleus; 8, Luschka recess; 9, superior fovea; 10, stria medullaris; 11, inferior fovea; 12, inferior cerebellar peduncle; 13, obex; 14, choroid plexus; IV, trochlear n rootlets; VII, facial colliculus; VIII, vestibular area; X, vagal trigone; XII, hypoglossal trigone; C, cuneate tubercle; G, gracile tubercle. **B. Circumventricular organs:** Epiphysis (pineal gland), hypophysis (median eminence and posterior pituitary gland), organum vasculosum of lamina terminalis, subcommissural organ, subfornical organ, area postrema. They are devoid of BBB except subcommissural organ. Area postrema is paired, located in the floor of the fourth ventricle toward the obex, between the vagal trigone and gracile tubercle; it has chemoreceptors for vomiting in response to circulating emetics like digitalis. II, optic n and chiasm; III, oculomotor n; IC, inferior colliculus; MB, mammillary body.

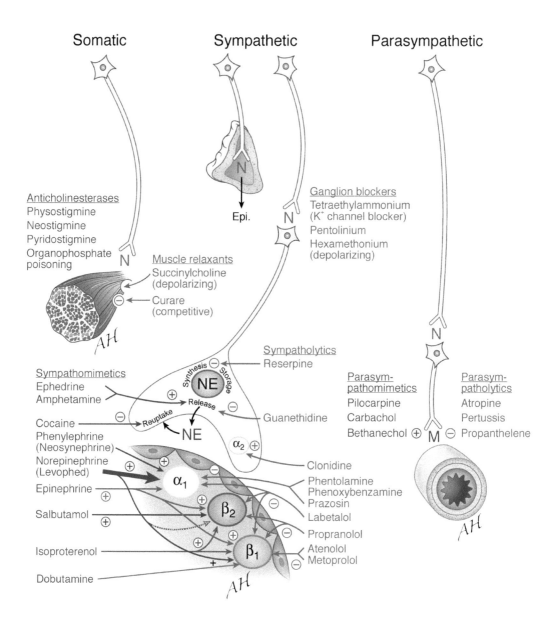

Somatic

Sympathetic

Parasympathetic

Epi.

Anticholinesterases
Physostigmine
Neostigmine
Pyridostigmine
Organophosphate
poisoning

Ganglion blockers
Tetraethylammonium
(K⁺ channel blocker)
Pentolinium
Hexamethonium
(depolarizing)

Muscle relaxants
Succinylcholine
(depolarizing)
Curare
(competitive)

Sympatholytics
Reserpine

Sympathomimetics
Ephedrine
Amphetamine

Synthesis   Storage

NE

Release

Cocaine

Reuptake

Guanethidine

Phenylephrine
(Neosynephrine)

NE

Norepinephrine
(Levophed)

α_2

Epinephrine

α_1

Clonidine

Phentolamine
Phenoxybenzamine
Prazosin

Salbutamol

β_2

Labetalol

Isoproterenol

β_1

Propranolol

Atenolol
Metoprolol

Dobutamine

Parasym-
pathomimetics
Pilocarpine
Carbachol
Bethanechol

Parasym-
patholytics
Atropine
Pertussis
Propanthelene

Fig. 25 Peripheral nervous system. somatic, sympathetic, and parasympathetic. Different stimulants are depicted in blue while inhibitors are depicted in red. Epi, epinephrine; M, muscarinic acetylcholine receptors; N, nicotinic acetylcholine receptors; NE, norepinephrine. Note that postganglionic sympathetic output to sweat glands utilizes muscarinic acetylcholine receptors. Of note β3 receptors exist in adipose tissue and play a role in lipolysis and thermogenesis. They also lower blood glucose. Copyright Amgad Hanna.

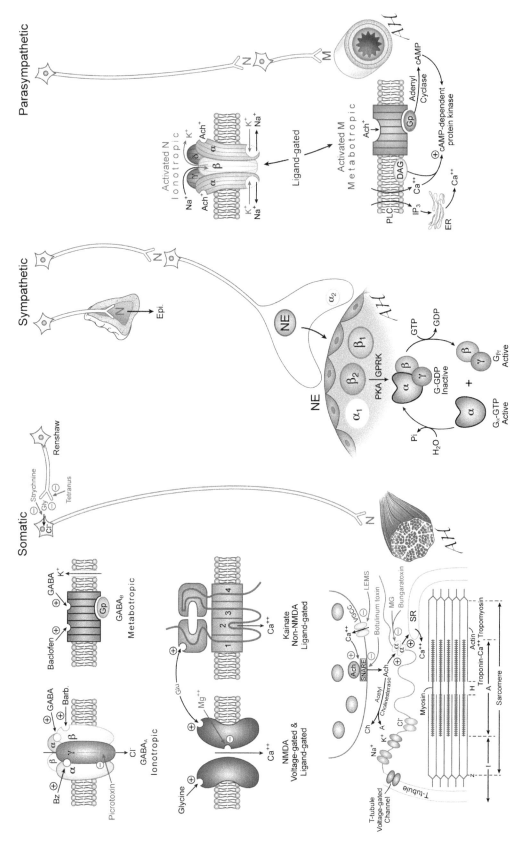

Fig. 26 Important receptors in the nervous system. In the CNS, γ-aminobutyric acid (GABA) and glutamate (Glu) receptors are common. $GABA_A$ is ionotropic, has five subunits (2α, 2β, 1γ); it can be activated by GABA, barbiturates (Barb), or benzodiazepines (Bz), thus opening a Cl^- channel in the center and causing Cl^- influx and hyperpolarization. $GABA_B$ is metabotropic, has seven transmembrane domains that activate G protein (Gp), resulting in K^+ efflux, inhibition of Ca^{++} influx, and hyperpolarization (neuronal inhibition). Glu receptors are either N-methyl-D-aspartate (NMDA) or *non*-NMDA (e.g., kainate). The former is voltage-gated and ligand-gated while the latter is ligand-gated only. They are both excitatory and cause Ca^{++} influx. In the spinal cord, Renshaw cells are inhibitory and utilize the neurotransmitter glycine (Gly). They are inhibited by tetanus (blocks Gly release) and strychnine (blocks Gly receptors) causing contractures. Nicotinic acetylcholine receptors (N) are found at the neuromuscular junction, the adrenal medulla stimulating release of epinephrine (Epi), sympathetic and parasympathetic ganglia. At the neuromuscular junction, Lambert–Eaton myasthenic syndrome (LEMS) is caused by inhibition of the release of acetylcholine (Ach) by antibodies blocking presynaptic voltage-gated calcium channels (VGCC). Botulinum toxin blocks the release of Ach by inhibiting SNARE (Soluble N-ethylmaleimide-sensitive factor attachment protein receptor). Bungaratoxin blocks Ach receptors. Myasthenia gravis (MG) is caused by antibodies against Ach receptors, muscle-specific tyrosine kinase (MuSK), or more rarely titin, lipoprotein-related protein receptor 4 (LRP4), or ryanodine receptors. Ach causes Ca^{++} release from the sarcoplasmic reticulum (SR). It is degraded by acetylcholinesterase into choline (Ch) and acetate (A). In the autonomic ganglia, N is composed of five subunits (2α, β, γ, δ), each one composed of four transmembrane domains. It is ionotropic, ligand-gated, and when activated opens a central pore and expands the holes in the lateral walls of the intracellular part causing Na^+ influx and K^+ efflux. Muscarinic Ach receptors (M) are found at the postganglionic parasympathetic and sympathetic endings to sweat glands. They are metabotropic, ligand-gated, and composed of seven transmembrane proteins that activate Gp. cAMP, cyclic adenosine monophosphate; DAG, diacyl glycerol; ER, endoplasmic reticulum; IP3, inositol triphosphate; PLC, phospholipase C. Norepinephrine (NE) is released from sympathetic nerve endings. It activates Gp through Gp receptor kinase (GPRK) or protein kinase A (PKA). GDP, guanosine diphosphate; GTP, guanosine triphosphate; Pi, inorganic phosphate. Copyright Amgad Hanna.

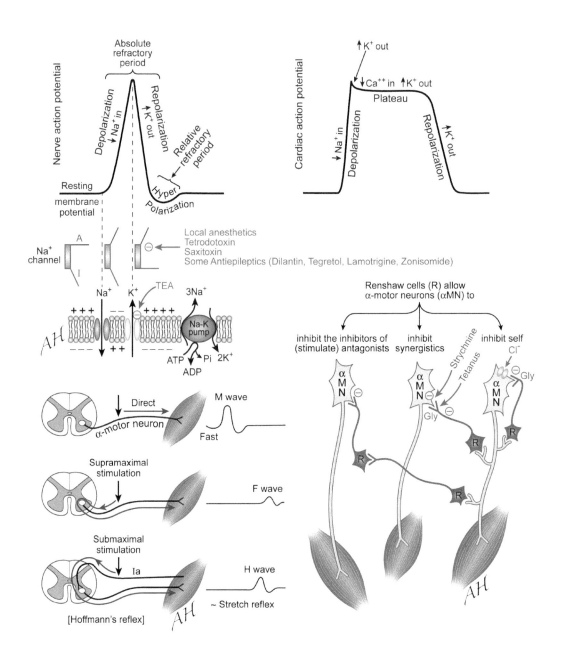

Fig. 27 Action potential. Nerve action potential (top left): During the resting state, the sodium channels are closed by the activation gate (A), while the inactivation gate (I) is open. During depolarization, both gates are open and sodium ions rush inside the cell. Repolarization occurs because the inactivation gate closes, while K^+ exits the cell. Tetrodotoxin, saxitoxin, local anesthetics, and some antiepileptics block Na^+ channels, while tetraethylammonium (TEA) inhibits K^+ channels. Pi, phosphate. Na-K pump restores a higher concentration of Na^+ outside the cell and K^+ inside the cell; it requires energy. Cardiac muscle action potential (top right) is characterized by a plateau phase where depolarization is slowed down by Ca^{++} influx. Ca^{++} is used for cardiac muscle contraction. EMG (bottom left) waves showing the H (Hoffmann) reflex, which is the electric equivalent of the stretch (myotatic) reflex, it results from submaximal stimulation. With supramaximal stimulation, antidromic transmission through the α-motor neuron results in the F wave. The M wave results from orthodromic stimulation of the α-motor neuron, thus directly stimulating the muscle with short latency. Renshaw cells (R, bottom right) moderate muscle contraction through feedback inhibition of the synergistic muscles and stimulation of antagonistic muscles. They utilize the neurotransmitter glycine (Gly), which increases Cl^- influx. Tetanus blocks glycine release and strychnine blocks glycine receptors causing muscle rigidity. Copyright Amgad Hanna.

Reproduced from *Source:* Vandenberg RJ, French CR, Barry PH, Shine J, Schofield PR. Antagonism of ligand-gated ion channel receptors: two domains of the glycine receptor alpha subunit form the strychnine-binding site. *Proc Natl Acad Sci USA* 1992 Mar 1; 89(5): 1765–1769

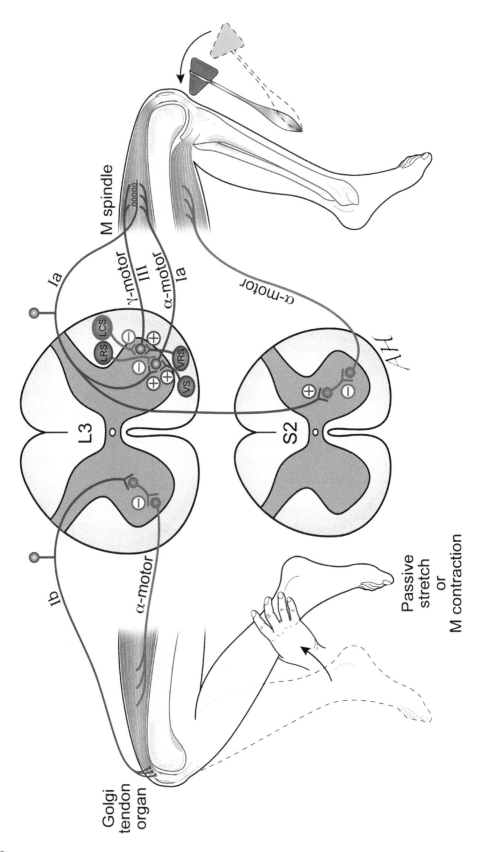

Fig. 28 Muscle tone and reflexes. Golgi tendon organ is stimulated by muscle contraction or strong passive stretch. Impulses travel through type Ib fibers to the dorsal root ganglion (DRG) then the spinal cord, to inhibit the corresponding muscle through a polysynaptic reflex. On the other hand, the patellar stretch (myotatic) reflex is monosynaptic: Stimulation of the patellar tendon with a reflex hammer causes acute stretch of the quadriceps tendon and stimulation of the muscle spindle. Impulse travels through Ia fibers to the DRG, to the spinal cord, then directly stimulate the α-motor neuron (Ia fibers) of the quadriceps. Collaterals are sent to inhibit the hamstrings. γ-motor neurons (III fibers) stimulate the muscle spindle to increase tone. Also, the ventral reticulospinal (VRS) and vestibulospinal (VS) tracts increase tone. The VS tract originates at the lateral vestibular (Deiter's) nucleus and is responsible for decerebrate rigidity. The lateral reticulospinal (LRS) and lateral corticospinal (LCS) tracts inhibit muscle tone. Loss of LCS inhibition is responsible for the spasticity associated with upper motor neuron lesions, e.g., hemiplegia or paraplegia. Of note, the muscle spindle also sends signals from primary annulospiral fibers. Copyright Amgad Hanna.

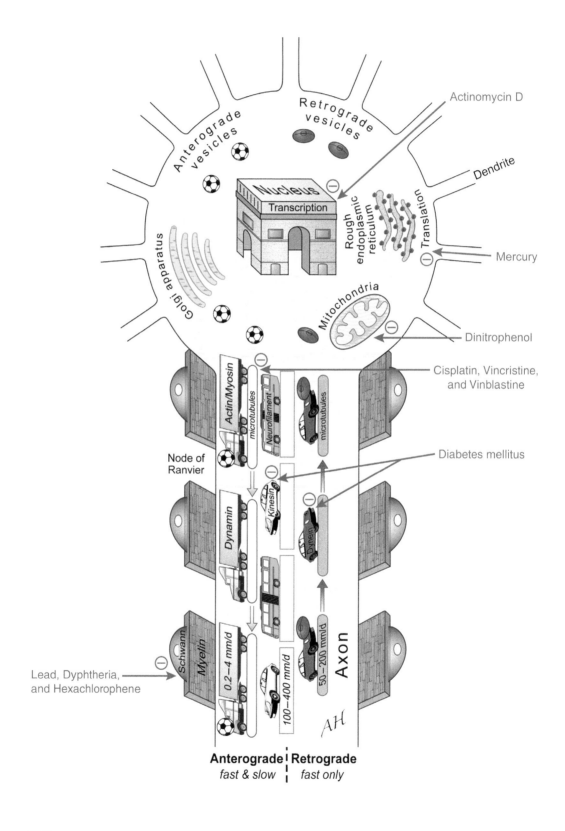

Fig. 29 Axonal transport. An axon is represented here by the Avenue des Champs-Élysées in Paris which stems out of Place Charles de Gualle-Étoile (cell body), with the Arc de Triomphe (nucleus) in its center. The dendrites are represented by the 11 other streets that stem from the same Place. Retrograde axonal transport is fast only (50–200 mm/d). The retrograde motor (Dynein) is represented by the red sports cars and the retrograde vesicles are represented by the rugby balls. The anterograde transport can be fast (100–400 mm/d) or slow (0.2–4 mm/d). The anterograde fast motor (Kinesin) is represented by the yellow sports cars, while the slow motors (Dynamin, actin, myosin) are the blue trucks. The soccer balls are the anterograde vesicles and the green buses are the neurofilaments. The buildings on the sides of the road represent Schwann cells and myelin. Microtubules (formed of α-tubulin and β-tubulin) form the skeleton of transport in both directions. Copyright Amgad Hanna.

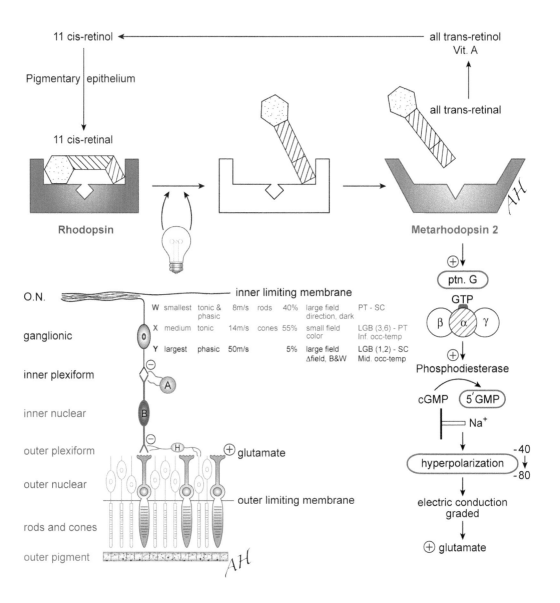

11 cis-retinol ← all trans-retinol Vit. A

Pigmentary epithelium

all trans-retinal

11 cis-retinal

Rhodopsin

Metarhodopsin 2

⊕ ptn. G

GTP

β   α   γ

⊕

Phosphodiesterase

cGMP   5′ GMP

Na⁺

hyperpolarization   -40 / -80

electric conduction graded

⊕ glutamate

O.N.   inner limiting membrane

W	smallest	tonic & phasic	8m/s	rods	40%	large field direction, dark	PT - SC
X	medium	tonic	14m/s	cones	55%	small field color	LGB (3,6) - PT Inf. occ-temp
Y	largest	phasic	50m/s		5%	large field Δfield, B&W	LGB (1,2) - SC Mid. occ-temp

ganglionic

O

inner plexiform

⊖   A

inner nuclear

B

outer plexiform

⊖   H   ⊕ glutamate

outer nuclear

outer limiting membrane

rods and cones

outer pigment

Fig. 30 Retina and vision. Layers of the retina and types of ganglion cells (bottom left). A, amacrine cells; B, bipolar cells; B&W, black-and-white vision; H, horizontal cells; Inf. occ-temp, inferior occipitotemporal cortex; LGB, lateral geniculate body; Mid. occ-temp, middle occipitotemporal cortex; PT, pretectum; SC, superior colliculus. Light converts rhodopsin to metarhodopsin 2, thus activating G protein (ptn. G), to convert cyclic guanosine monophosphate (cGMP) into 5′ guanosine monophosphate (5′GMP), thus decreasing Na$^+$ conductance and hyperpolarization. This results in graded electrical conduction. Copyright Amgad Hanna.

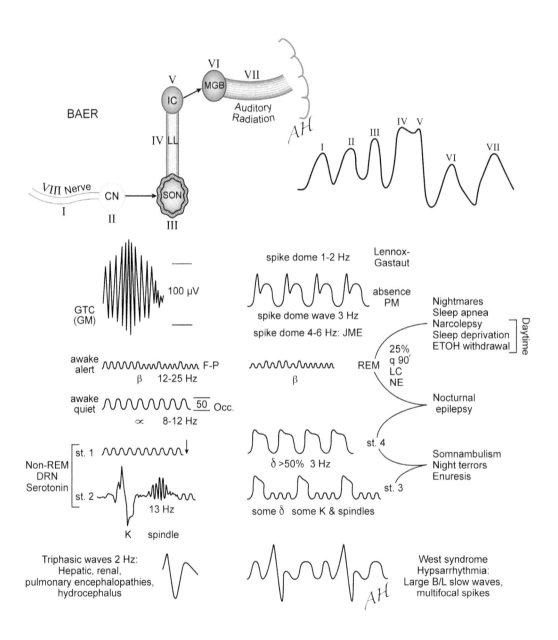

BAER

VIII Nerve

spike dome 1-2 Hz — Lennox-Gastaut

spike dome wave 3 Hz — absence PM

spike dome 4-6 Hz: JME

GTC (GM)

100 μV

awake alert — β 12-25 Hz — F-P

awake quiet — α 8-12 Hz — 50 Occ.

Non-REM DRN Serotonin

st. 1

st. 2 — 13 Hz

K — spindle

β

REM — 25% q 90′ LC NE

δ >50% 3 Hz — st. 4

some δ some K & spindles — st. 3

Nightmares
Sleep apnea
Narcolepsy
Sleep deprivation
ETOH withdrawal — Daytime

Nocturnal epilepsy

Somnambulism
Night terrors
Enuresis

Triphasic waves 2 Hz:
Hepatic, renal,
pulmonary encephalopathies,
hydrocephalus

West syndrome
Hypsarrhythmia:
Large B/L slow waves,
multifocal spikes

Fig. 31 Brain waves. Brainstem auditory evoked response (BAER) consists of seven waves: I, cochlear n (VIII); II, cochlear nuclei (CN); III, superior olivary nucleus (SON); IV, lateral lemniscus (LL); V, inferior colliculus (IC); VI, medial geniculate body (MGB); and VII, auditory radiation. Waves IV and V are the most sensitive, significant change occurs with 50-60% loss of amplitude or > 1 msec increase in latency. Generalized tonic–clonic (GTC) seizures or grand mal (GM) seizures are characterized by high-frequency large-amplitude (100 µV) spikes. Spike-dome waves at 1–2 Hz are seen in Lennox–Gastaut syndrome, at 3 Hz in petit mal (PM) or absence seizures, and at 4–6 Hz in juvenile myoclonic epilepsy (JME). B/L, bilateral; DRN, dorsal raphe nucleus; F-P, frontoparietal; LC, locus ceruleus; NE, norepinephrine; non-REM, non-rapid eye movement sleep; Occ, occipital; REM, rapid eye movement sleep. During acute focal destructive brain lesions (stroke, abscess, herpes encephalitis) periodic lateralized epileptiform discharges (PLEDs) can be observed. Generalized periodic epileptiform discharges (GPEDs) are seen in metabolic, infectious disease, subacute sclerosing panencephalitis (SSPE), and Creutzfeldt–Jakob disease (CJD). Copyright Amgad Hanna.

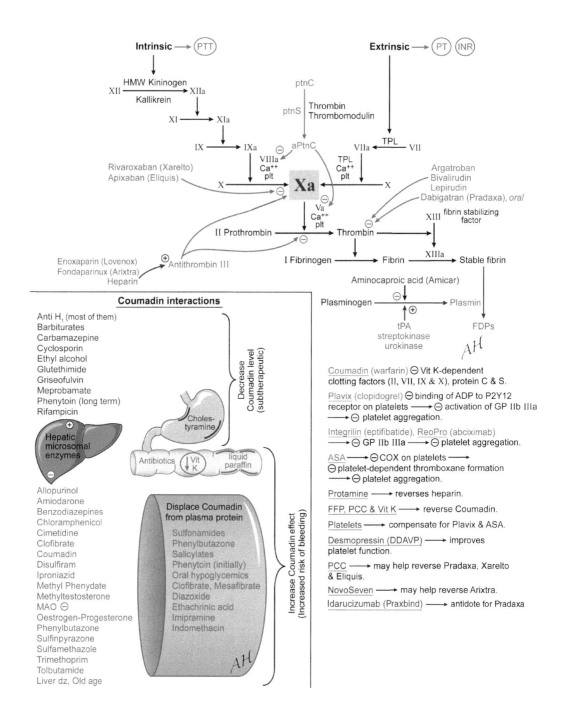

Fig. 32 Coagulation cascades and drugs affecting blood coagulation. ADP, adenosine diphosphate; ASA, acetyl salicylic acid; COX, cyclo-oxygenase; dz, disease; FDPs, fibrin degradation products; FFP, fresh frozen plasma; GP IIb IIIa, glycoprotein IIbIIIa; HMW, high molecular weight; INR, international normalized ratio; MAO ⊖, monoamine oxidase inhibitors; PCC (Kcentra), prothrombin complex concentrate; plt, platelets; PT, prothrombin time depends on the extrinsic pathway; ptn, protein; PTT, partial thromboplastin time, affected by the intrinsic pathway; tPA, tissue plasminogen activator; TPL, tissue thromboplastin. Cholestyramine decreases Coumadin absorption. Liquid paraffin decreases absorption of vitamin K (Vit K). Idarucizumab (Praxbind) is an antibody that can bind and reverse Pradaxa. Copyright Amgad Hanna. Published with permission.

Section III. Tables

Table 1. Nerve fibers

Fiber	AKA	Velocity (m/s)	Function
Ia	A α	120	α motor neuron (← stretch [myotatic] reflex ←) muscle spindle (1ary, annulospiral)
Ib	A α	120	Golgi tendon organ (→ + Renshaw C → – α motor neuron)
II	A β, γ	30–70	fine touch, pressure, vibration, muscle spindle (2ary, flower-spray)
III	A δ	5–30	pain (sharp), temp (cold), light touch, γ motor neuron (→ + muscle spindle → increase tone)
IV Unmyelinated	C	<2	pain (burning), temp (hot, cold), light touch (tickle), itch, sympathetic postganglionic

Table 2. Nerve receptors

Receptor	Location	Sensation	Adaptation	Receptive field	Fibers
Meissner's corpuscles	Dermal papillae of fingertips, lips	Touch, vibration	Rapid (phasic)	Small	II
Pacinian corpuscles	Deep	Vibration		Large	II
Hair end organs	Hair follicles	Touch			
Ruffini end organs	Deep	Heavy touch and pressure	Slow (tonic)	Large	II
Merkel's discs	Dermal papillae	Touch and pressure		Small	II
Free nerve endings		Light touch, pressure, pain, temp, tickle, itch		Small	III, IV

Table 3. Intrafusal muscle fibers (m spindle)

Type	Nuclear bag	Nuclear chain
Size	Larger	Smaller
Firing	Dynamic	Static
	Tonic, variable	Tonic
Receptors	Primary (annulospiral)	Primary (annulospiral) and secondary (flower-spray)
Location	Central	Eccentric
Fibers	Ia	II
Velocity (m/s)	120	30–70

Table 4. Types of skeletal muscle fibers

	Type I	Type II
Twitch (contraction)	Slow	Fast
Fatigability	Slow	Fast
Metabolism	Aerobic	Anaerobic
Lactic acid production	Low	High
Mitochondrial content	High	Low
Capillary bed	Extensive	Limited
Main fuel	Triglycerides	Glycogen
Sports	Endurance	Strength

Table 5. Blood signals on MRI

Stage	T1 MRI	T2 MRI	Blood product
Hyperacute (hr)	I	B	OxyHb
Acute	I	D	DeoxyHb
Early subacute (3–14 d)	B	D	MetHb, intracellular
Late subacute (>2 wk)	B	B	MetHb, extracellular
Chronic	D	D	Ferritin, hemosiderin

Abbreviations: I, isointense; B, bright (hyperintense); D, dark (hypointense); Hb, hemoglobin.

Table 6. Genetic alterations in glioblastoma (GBM)

Primary GBM	Secondary GBM
LOH 10q (70%)	**LOH 10q (63%)**
EGFR ++ (36%)	EGFR ++ (8%)
p16^{INK4a} deletion (31%)	p16^{INK4a} deletion (19%)
TP53 mutation (28%)	***TP53 mutation (65%)***
PTEN mutation (25%)	PTEN mutation (4%)

Abbreviations: EGFR ++, epidermal growth factor receptor amplification; LOH 10q, loss of heterozygosity of the long arm of chromosome 10; p16^{INK4a}, a tumor suppressor protein on the short arm of chromosome 9; PTEN, phosphatase and tension homolog, a tumor suppressor on the long arm of chromosome 10; TP53, tumor protein 53, a tumor suppressor gene on the short arm of chromosome 17.

Sources: Ohgaki H, Kleihues P. The definition of primary and secondary glioblastoma. *Clin Cancer Res* 2013 Feb 15;19(4):764–772; Ohgaki H, Kleihues P. Genetic pathways to primary and secondary glioblastoma. *Am J Pathol* 2007 May;170(5):1445–1453; Ohgaki H, Kleihues P. Population-based studies on incidence, survival rates, and genetic alterations in astrocytic and oligodendroglial gliomas. *J Neuropathol Exp Neurol* 2005 Jun;64(6):479–489

Note: Secondary GBM occurs in younger patients and has better prognosis. *O-6-methylguanine-DNA methyltransferase* (MGMT) methylation indicates better prognosis and increased efficacy of temozolomide. *Isocitrate dehydrogenase 1 (IDH1)* mutation has better prognosis. Co-deletion of *1p19q* is good prognostic predictor in oligodendrogliomas. Of note in medulloblastomas, WNT has the best prognosis and group 3 has the worst.

Table 7. Different rosette structures associated with brain tumors

Rosette	Description	Tumor
Pseudorosette	Central vessel	Ependymoma
Flexner–Wintersteiner	Central canal	Pineoblastoma, retinoblastoma, ependymoma
Homer–Wright	No central vessel or canal	Medulloblastoma, PNET
	Very large	Pineocytoma

Table 8. Craniopharyngioma subtypes

Adamantinomatous	Papillary
Children	Adults
Calcifications	Rare
Cysts	Infrequent
Keratinized ghost cells	No
Squamous cells surrounded by columnar cells	Squamous cells
Worse prognosis	Better prognosis

Table 9. Developmental disorders of the nervous system

Gestational age	Event	Pathology
3–4 wks	Primary neurulation	Myelomeningocele
4–5 wks	Secondary neurulation	Myelocystocele (abnormal disjunction)
		Dermal sinus
		Diastematomyelia
5–10 wks	Ventral induction	Holoprosencephaly
2–5 mo	Migration	Corpus callosum agenesis, colpocephaly
		Cavum septum pellucidum
		Polymicrogyria, pachygyria, lissencephaly
		Megalencephaly
		Schizencephaly, porencephaly

Table 10. Different inclusion bodies in health and disease

Inclusion bodies	Disease	Comments
Lewy	Parkinson's	Intracytoplasmic
Hirano	Alzheimer's	Intracytoplasmic & extracellular
Bunina	ALS	Intracytoplasmic
Lafora	Lafora's	Intracytoplasmic
Pick	Pick's	Intracytoplasmic
Ne**gr**i	**R**abies	Intracytoplasmic, Pu**r**kinje cells (cerebellum), hippocampus
Cowdry type A	Herpes simplex	Intranuclear
Cowdry type A	Cytomegalovirus	Intranuclear & intracytoplasmic
Inclusion bodies	Measles	Intranuclear & intracytoplasmic
Russell	Multiple myeloma	Intracytoplasmic immunoglobulin in plasma cells
Marinesco		Normal in brain stem melanocytes
Herring		Neurosecretory terminals in posterior pituitary

Source: Krishnan B, Thiagarajan P. Images in hematology. Myeloma with Russell bodies. *Am J Hematol* 2005 Jan;78(1):79

Table 11. Familial tumors

Syndrome	Chromosome	Inheritance	Neoplasms
Von Hippel–Lindau (VHL)	3	Autosomal dominant	Hemangioblastoma, renal cell carcinoma, pheochromocytoma
Turcot	5	Autosomal dominant	Medull**o**blastoma, gli**o**blastoma, **colo**n p**o**lyp**o**sis or aden**o**car**c**in**o**ma
Gorlin	9	Autosomal dominant	Medull**o**blastoma, meningioma, basal cell nevus syndrome
Tuberous sclerosis	9 (TSC1, hamartin) & 16 (TSC2, tuberin)	Autosomal dominant	Subependymal giant cell astrocytoma (SEGA), cardiac rhabdomyoma, pancreatic adenoma, renal angiolipoma, cysts (lung, liver, and spleen), facial angiofibroma (adenoma sebaceum), subungual fibroma (Koenen tumor), ash leaf spots
Cowden	10 (PTEN mutation)	Autosomal dominant	Lhermitte–Duclos disease, breast, uterine, and thyroid carcinoma
Multiple endocrine neoplasia (MEN) 1 (Wermer's syndrome)	11	Autosomal dominant	**P**ituitary adenoma, **p**arathyroid adenoma, and **p**ancreatic islet tumors
Li–Fraumeni	17 (TP53)	Autosomal dominant	Astrocytoma, sarcoma, breast carcinoma
Neurofibromatosis 1 (NF1)	17	Autosomal dominant	Neurofibromas, plexiform neurofibroma, malignant peripheral nerve sheath tumor (MPNST), optic n glioma, Lisch nodules (iris), axillary freckling, café au lait spots, bony dysplasia
Neurofibromatosis 2 (NF2)	22	Autosomal dominant	Schwannoma, meningioma, ependymoma, posterior subcapsular cataract

Table 12. Congenital metabolic disorders

Disease	Inheritance	Enzyme	Labs	Clinical Picture
I—Aminoacidopathies				
Phenylketonuria	AR 12	Phenylalanine hydroxylase	Increased serum phenylalanine, increased urine phenyl pyruvic acid	Fair-skinned, blue eyes, musty odor
Homocystinuria	AR	Cystathionine synthetase	Defective methionine metabolism	Strokes, **MR**, tall, thin, lens dislocation, arachnodactyly, Tx: B6, B12, decreased methionine, increased cysteine intake
Maple syrup urine disease	AR	Decreased branching chain aa catabolism		Death by 4 wks unless leucine, isoleucine, and valine intake is limited
II—Sphingolipidoses (lysosomal storage Dz)				
(A) Gangliosidoses [ganglioside = ceramide + sialic acid]				
GM1	AR	β-galactosidase		***Cherry-red*** macula, **HSM**, bone abnormalities, dysmorphic face, contractures
Sandhoff's Dz (GM2)	AR	Hexosaminidase A & B		***Cherry-red*** macula, **HSM**
Tay–Sachs Dz (GM2)	AR	Hexosaminidase A		***Cherry-red*** macula, micro or **Macrocephaly**, blindness in children, ataxia in young adults, Ashkenasi Jews
(B) Cerebrosides [cerebroside = ceramide + hexose]				
Gaucher's Dz	AR	Glucocerebrosidase	Gaucher Cs: wrinkled tissue paper appearance	Non-neuropathic, **HSM**, lungs, anemia, thrombocytopenia, Ashkenasi Jews
(C) Sphingomyelins [sphingomyelin = ceramide + choline P]				
Niemann–Pick Dz	AR	Sphingomyelinase	Foam Cs	***Cherry-red*** macula, **HSM**, **MR**, supranuclear paresis of vertical gaze, Ashkenasi Jews
(D) Ceramides [ceramide = sphingosine + LCFA]				
Fabry's Dz	XR	α-galactosidase A		**C**orneal opacities, **C**erebrovascular occlusions (non-cortical neurons), PN (pain, dysesthesia, wea**k**ness), **C**AD, HTN, **k**idney insufficiency, s**k**in angiokeratomas
III—Mucopolysaccharidoses				
Hurler's Dz (MPS IH)	AR	α-L-iduronidase	Ur dermatan s, Zebra bodies	**MR,** worst, gargoyle face, thick meninges, SC compression, corneal opacities, conduction deafness, cardiac Dz, **HSM**
Scheie's S (MPS IS)	AR	α-L-iduronidase	Ur dermatan s, Zebra bodies	Best, mild form of Hurler, CTS, no MR

(continued)

225

Table 12. Congenital metabolic disorders (*Continued*)

Disease	Inheritance	Enzyme	Labs	Clinical Picture
Hunter's S (MPS II)	XR	Iduronate-2-sulfatase	Ur dermatan s	Skin pebbling, no or mild MR
Sanfilippo's S (MPS III)	AR	Heparan sulfatase	Ur heparan s	**MR**
Morquio's S (MPS IV)	AR	N-acetyl-galactos-amine-6-sulfatase & β-galactosidase	Ur keratan s	Odontoid hypoplasia, thick cervical dura, myelopathy, dwarfism, osteoporosis, ligamentous laxity, no MR
Maroteaux–Lamy S (MPS VI)	AR	Arylsulfatase B (N-acetylgalactos-amine-4-sulfatase)	Ur dermatan s	Cervical myelopathy, **HSM**, no MR
Sly's S (MPS VII)	AR	β-glucuronidase	Ur heparan, dermatan, and chon-droitin s	**MR**, corneal clouding, **HSM**, bony changes

IV—Leukodystrophies = dysmyelinating Dz MR in all

Disease	Inheritance	Enzyme	Labs	Clinical Picture
Krabbe's Dz	AR	Galactocerebroside β-galactosidase (lysosomal)	Globoid cells, spares U fibers	**MR**, microcephaly, PN
Metachromatic leukodystrophy	AR 22	Arylsulfatase A (lysosomal)	Hirsch–Peiffer reaction (tissue turns brown with acidic cresyl violet), spares U fibers	**MR**, PN, **HSM**, kidney insufficiency
Adrenoleukody-strophy	XR	Defect lipid oxidation in peroxisomes: ATP-binding transporter ptn, VLCFA accumulation	Spares U fibers, parieto-occipital cavitation	**MR**, adrenal insufficiency, bronze skin, decreased vision and hearing
Pelizaeus–Merzbacher Dz	XR	Defect synthesis of proteolipid lipoprotein, inducing apoptosis in oligodendroglia	Tigroid pattern (MRI), cerebellar involvement	**MR**, nystagmus, ataxia, spasticity
Canavan's Dz	AR	Deficiency N-acetyl-aspartoacylase	Affects U fibers, spongy WM, occipital lobes, markedly enlarged mitochondria, N-acetyl aspartic aciduria	**MR, Macrocephaly**, blindness, Ashkenasi Jews

Table 12. Congenital metabolic disorders (*Continued*)

Disease	Inheritance	Enzyme	Labs	Clinical Picture
Alexander's Dz		GFAP disorder; astrocytes	Frontal lobes, Rosenthal fibers	**MR, Macrocephaly**, Sz
Sudanophyllic leukodystrophy				**MR**, blindness, spasticity
Cockayne's syndrome		DNA repair disorder		CNS and PN demyelination, cataract, dwarfism
V—Others				
Leigh's Dz	AR	Mitochondrial dysfunction (Cytochrome C oxidase)	Bilateral symmetric spongiform degeneration of BG, thalamus, brain stem, and SC. Demyelinating PN	Sz, ophthalmoplegia, decreased tone
Zellweger's syndrome	AR	Decreased liver peroxisomes, LCFA accumulation		Cerebro-hepato-renal syndrome
Lowe's syndrome	XR			Oculo-cerebro-renal syndrome
Lesch–Nyhan Dz	XR	Decreased HGPRT (Hypoxanthine Guanine Phospho-Ribosyl transferase)	Uric acid accumulation	Self-mutilation, choreoathetosis
Menke's kinky hair Dz	XR	Decreased Cu absorption from GI	Diffuse loss of neurons	**MR**, colorless brittle hair, Sz, intracranial aneurysm, tortuous abdominal viscera
Carnithine deficiency		Inability to use LCFA		Mild weakness

Abbreviations: aa, amino acids; AD, autosomal dominant; AR, autosomal recessive; BG, basal ganglia; CAD, coronary artery disease; CNS, central nervous system; CTS, carpal tunnel syndrome; Dz, disease; GI, gastrointestinal tract; HSM, hepatosplenomegaly; HTN, hypertension; LCFA, long-chain fatty acids; MR, mental retardation; PN, peripheral neuropathy; Ptn, protein; S, syndrome; s sulfate; SC, spinal cord; Sz, seizures; Tx, treatment; Ur, urinary; VLCFA, very long-chain fatty acids; WM, white matter; XR, X-linked recessive.

Table 13. Neuropathies and myopathies

Disease	Inheritance	Enzyme	Labs	Clinical Picture
Hereditary neuropathies (onion bulb)				
Charcot–Marie–Tooth (peroneal m atrophy)	AD		DRG, posterior column, AHC, demyelination and remyelination	Peroneal m atrophy, NL CSF
Dejerine–Sottas Dz	AD		Demyelination and remyelination	Enlarged nontender ulnar, median, radial, and peroneal nn, claw hands and feet, symmetric
Refsum's Dz	AR	Phytanic acid oxidase		PN: LE, symmetric, S=M, *retinitis pigmentosum*, hearing loss, and cardiomyopathy
Degenerative neuropathies (motor neuron Dz) (sensory and bladder intact)				
ALS (Lou Gehrig's)	AD 21	Cu/Zn superoxide dismutase mutation	Bunina bodies (intracellular). EMG: fasciculations & fibrillation. MRI: increased flair signal of corticospinal tracts bilaterally	UMNL & LMNL, fasciculations & atrophy (tongue, face, and hands), hyper- or hyporeflexia, Babinski, **Tx: Relotec (antiglutamate)**
SMA-1 (Werdnig–Hoffmann Dz)	AR 5q mostly			AHC + XII, most common, worst, acute infantile
SMA-2	AR 5q			AHC + XII, chronic infantile
SMA-3 (Wohlfart–Kugelberg–Welander)	AR 5q			AHC + XII, chronic childhood
Muscular dystrophies (MD)				
Duchenne's MD (most common MD in children)	XR	Decreased dystrophin	**Incr CK +++**, m fiber necrosis and regeneration	atrophy shoulder and pelvic girdles, calf pseudohypertrophy, + Gower's test, CHF, respiratory infections, **MR** occasionally, **Tx Prednisone**
Becker's MD	XR	Abnormal dystrophin		Less severe than Duchenne
Emery–Dreifuss	XR			Early contractures of elbow flexors, calf, and neck extensors, cardiomyopathy
Limb–girdle MD	AR	Mutation in dystrophin-associated glycoprotein (sarcoglycan)	m fiber hypertrophy with splitting	Pseudohypertrophy 33%, CHF

Table 13. Neuropathies and myopathies (*Continued*)

Disease	Inheritance	Enzyme	Labs	Clinical Picture
Myotonic MD (most common MD in adults)	AD 19	CTG trinucleotide repetition (>50 copies)	Ring fibers. EMG: "Dive bomber" frequency	Face then distal extremities, **MR**, dysrhythmias, cataract, endocrinopathies, frontal baldness, **Tx: Quinine, procainamide, dilantin**
Facioscapulo-humeral MD (Landouzi–Dejerine)	AD 4		Chronic inflammatory cells in m	SN hearing loss
Oculopharyngeal MD	AD 14	GCG repeats (>8–13)	Tubulofilamentous intranuclear inclusions, amyloid	Ptosis, dysphagia
Glycogen storage Dz				
*M*cArdle's Dz	AR 11	*M*yophosphorylase deficiency	**Increased CK,** LDH in serum, myoglobinuria	Myalgia, cramping, stiffness, only symptomatic with activity
Phosphofructokinase deficiency	AR 12			Similar to McArdle's
Pompe's Dz	AR 17	Acid maltase deficiency	Glycogen in liver, heart, skeletal m, and motor neuron	Hepatomegaly, cardiorespiratory death
Inflammatory myopathies				
Dermatomyositis		B cell-mediated, complement	Perifascicular m degeneration and atrophy, perivascular B-lymphocytes	Butterfly rash on face, Gottron's papules at knuckles, angiopathy of skin, n, m, intestines, Raynaud's phenomenon (30%), CA (10%), **Tx: steroids**
Polymyositis		T cell-mediated (CD 8+; cytotoxic)	Necrosis and phagocytosis of individual m fibers	Painless, symmetric, proximal > distal weakness, CA (10%) anti Jo-1, increased ESR, ANA, **CK** and urinary myoglobin. EMG: MUPs small amplitude & short duration, fibrillation potential, and sharp waves. **Tx: steroids**
Inclusion body myositis		Autoimmune caused by virus or prion	Intranuclear inclusions	Painless, progressive LE weakness, steroid-resistant, 60-y-o males
Others				
Mitochondrial myopathies*	Maternal mitochondria	Large subsarcolemmal mitochondria	Red-ragged m fibers (trichrome stain), EM: Parking lot inclusions (mitochondria)	Retinal, ocular, and cardiac abnormalities

*MELAS: Myopathy, encephalopathy, lactic acidosis, and strokes; MERRF: Myoclonus, epilepsy, and red-ragged fibers; MNGIE: Mitochondrial, neuro, gastro-intestinal encephalopathy; Luft's Dz, Leigh's Dz

(continued)

Table 13. Neuropathies and myopathies (*Continued*)

Disease	Inheritance	Enzyme	Labs	Clinical Picture
Kearns–Sayre syndrome	AD	Mitochondrial DNA, non-maternally inherited	Increased serum pyruvate, spongy brain	Progressive external ophthalmoplegia, *retinitis pigmentosum*, cardiac conduction defects
Familial periodic paralysis	AD	Genetic defect coding for Ca in m fiber membranes	Low K+	Intermittent episodes of paralysis, caused by hyperthyroidism, cold weather, exercise, glucose, NaCl, **Tx: KCl, carbonic anhydrase inhibitors (dichlorphenamide), low NaCl, avoid carbohydrates**
Acute intermittent porphyria	AD	Defective porphobilinogen deaminase	Increased urinary δ-ALA and porphobilinogen, urine turns **dark** as it oxidizes	PN severe, symmetric, M>S, + autonomic, abdominal pain, Sz, psychiatric issues, **Tx: hematin**
Malignant hyperthermia	AD 19q	Ryanodine receptor mutation	Increased Ca++ release from sarcoplasmic reticulum, **increased CK**, hyperkalemia, myoglobinuria	Halothane and succinylcholine, fever, rigidity, hyperventilation, tachycardia, dysrhythmia, HTN, hypotension, **Tx: dantrolene**
Central core Dz	AD 19q	Ryanodine receptor mutation		

Abbreviations: AD, autosomal dominant; AHC, anterior horn cell; ALA, aminolevulinic acid; ANA, antinuclear antibody; AR, autosomal recessive; CA, cancer; CHF, congestive heart failure; CK, creatine kinase; DRG, dorsal root ganglion; Dz, disease; EM, electron microscopy; HTN, hypertension; LDH, lactate dehydrogenase; LE, lower extremities; LMNL, lower motor neuron lesion; m, muscle; M, motor; MR, mental retardation; MUP, motor unit potential; n, nerve; NL, normal; PN, peripheral neuropathy; S, sensory; SMA, spinal muscle atrophy; SN, sensory-neural; Sz, seizures; Tx, treatment; UMNL, upper motor neuron lesion; XR, X-linked recessive.

Table 14. Neurodegenerative diseases

Disease	Genetic	Onset (age; yrs)	Incidence/ Gender	Clinical Picture	Pathological	Survival (yrs)–treatment
Alzheimer's		80	1/10	Memory loss	Neurofibrillary tangles (tau ptn), neuritic plaques (β-amyloid), Hirano bodies, decreased Ach output to cerebral cortex	
Pick's		40–60	F	Frontal dysfunction	Pick bodies	2–5
Huntington's	AD-4, CAG repeats	30	1/10,000	Chorea	Caudate atrophy (box-car ventricles), decreased Ach in striatum	15–30 Haloperidol
Wilson's	AR-13	10–30	M	Hepatolenticular degeneration, *Kayser–Fleischer* ring in cornea	Opalski cells, Alzheimer II astrocytes, decreased serum Cu and ceruloplasmin, increased urinary Cu. Serum free (unbound) Cu can be elevated.	Tetrathio-molybdate, penicillamine, B6, Zn, decrease Cu intake
Steele–Richardson–Olszewski (progressive supranuclear palsy)		50–60	M	Decreased intellect, vision, speech, and abnormal gait. Rigidity, pseudobulbar palsy, vertical gaze palsy, opticokinetic nystagmus, decreased oculo-cephalic reflexes	Atrophy of superior colliculus, STN, SN, and GP	1–12
Parkinson's		40–50	1%, M	Bradykinesia, rigidity, resting tremor	Lewy bodies, decreased melanin and neurons in SN (decreased dopamine output), LC, and DNX	80% at 10 yrs
Diffuse Lewy body				= Parkinson + frontal atrophy (dementia)		
Striatonigral degeneration		50		= Parkinson – Lewy bodies		
Shy–Drager	Parkinson-plus	50–60		= Parkinson – Lewy bodies + autonomic dysfunction		7, DA resistant
Olivo-ponto-cerebellar atrophy	Parkinson-plus	15		Ataxia, Parkinson picture	Atrophy of inferior olive, pons, middle cerebellar peduncle, and cerebellum (multisystem atrophy)	DA resistant
Hallervorden–Spatz		Late childhood		Extrapyramidal, corticospinal, dementia,	Fe deposition in SN and GP → brown and atrophic. hypodense BG on CT	Early adulthood
Acquired hepato-cerebral degeneration			1% of liver cirrhosis patients	Parkinsonism and cerebellar signs. Occurs also with TPN (Mn)	Increased ammonia, portosystemic shunts, hyperintense GP (T1-MRI)	
Friedreich's ataxia	AR-9	<20		Diabetes mellitus, cardiomegaly	Degeneration of post erior columns, corticospinal, DRG, spinocerebellar, inferior olive, cerebellum, and cranial n nuclei (VIII, X, XII)	Mid-30s

Abbreviations: AD, autosomal dominant; AR, autosomal recessive; BG, basal ganglia; Cu, copper; DA, dopa; DNX, dorsal nucleus of vagus n; DRG, dorsal root ganglion; Fe, iron; GP, globus pallidus; LC, locus ceruleus; Mn, manganese; ptn, protein; SN, substantia nigra; STN, subthalamic nucleus; TPN, total parenteral nutrition; Zn, zinc.

Table 15. Multiple cranial nerve syndromes (skull base)

Syndrome	Cranial nerves
Vernet	IX, X, XI
Collet–Sicard	IX, X, XI, XII
Villaret	IX, X, XI, XII, Sympathetic, ± VII
Tapia	VII, X, XII, ± Sympathetic
Schmidt	X, XI
Garcin	Progressive, unilateral, pan-cranial neuropathy
Gradenigo (petrous apex)	VI, retro-ocular pain, ear discharge
Tolosa–Hunt (painful ophthalmoplegia)	III, IV, V$_1$, VI, periorbital pain
Ramsay Hunt (Herpes Zoster of the geniculate ganglion)	VII, VIII, pain, and vesicles in the external auditory canal

Table 16. Paraneoplastic syndromes

Antibody	Clinical Picture	Neoplasm associated
Anti-amphiphysin, gephyrin	Stiff-man (Moersch–Woltman) syndrome	Breast, when caused by anti-GAD is non-paraneoplastic
Anti-bipolar cells, anti-recoverin	Melanoma-associated retinopathy (MAR) and cancer-associated retinopathy (CAR)	Melanoma, small cell lung
Anti-H*u*	Peripheral ne*u*ropathy, limbic encephalopathy	Small cell l*u*ng, lymphoma
Anti-*Jo*	Polymyositis	Crypt*o*genic fibrosing alveolitis (non-paraneoplastic)
Anti-MA2	Brain s*t*em, limbic encephalitis	Lung, testis
Anti-*Ri*	Opsoclonus	B*r*east
Anti-*Ta*	Brain s*t*em and limbic encephali*tis*	*Test*icular
Anti-T*r*	Ce*r*ebellum, ante*r*ior ho*r*n cells	Hodgkin's
Anti-VGCC	Lambert–Eaton myasthenic syndrome	Small cell lung, gastrointestinal
Anti-Y*o*	Cerebellum	*O*vary, breast

Abbreviation: VGCC, voltage-gated calcium channels.

Table 17. Spinal AVMs

Types	Etiology	Age	Flow	Pressure	Location	Presentation
I—Dural AVF	Acquired	40–70	H	L	Nerve root, dorsal, lower thoracic	Venous hypertension (Foix–Alajouanine syndrome)
II—Glomus AVM	Congenital	Young	H	H	Intramedullary, dorsal, cervical	Hemorrhage
III—Juvenile AVM			H	H	Intramedullary & extramedullary	Hemorrhage, vascular steal
IV—Intradural extramedullary AVF		20–50	H	L	Intradural extramedullary, anterior, conus	Venous hypertension

Abbreviations: AVF, arteriovenous fistula; H, high; L, low.

Table 18. Borden's classification of cranial dural AVF

Type	Venous drainage
I	Dural sinus
II	Dural sinus + retrograde subarachnoid
III	Retrograde subarachnoid (highest risk of hemorrhage)

Table 19. Classification of caroticocavernous fistulae (CCF)

Type	Arterial connection to cavernous sinus
A	ICA, direct
B	ICA, meningeal branches
C	ECA, meningeal branches
D	(ICA + ECA), meningeal branches

Abbreviations: ICA, internal carotid artery; ECA, external carotid artery.

Table 20. Spetzler–Martin grading system for cranial AVMs

Size	<3 cm	1
	3–6	2
	>6 cm	3
Eloquent brain	No	0
	Yes	1
Deep venous drainage	No	0
	Yes	1

Table 21. Modified Hardy's classification of pituitary tumors

		0	Intrasellar
I	Sella normal or focally expanded	A	Suprasellar
II	Sella enlarged	B	Anterior recess of third ventricle
III	Sellar floor breach	C	Displaces floor of third ventricle
IV	Sellar floor destruction	D	Intradural spread (frontal, temporal)
V	CSF or blood-borne spread	E	Extradural spread (cavernous sinus)

Table 22. Clinical grading of subarachnoid hemorrhage

Hunt and Hess	Clinical Picture	WFNS	GCS	Motor deficits
I	Mild headache	I	15	−
II	Severe headache, cranial n deficits	II	13–14	−
III	Lethargy	III	13–14	+
IV	Hemiparesis, stupor	IV	7–12	+/−
V	Decerebrate rigidity	V	3–6	+/−

Abbreviations: GCS, Glasgow coma scale; WFNS, World Federation of Neurosurgical Societies.

Table 23. Fisher grading of subarachnoid hemorrhage (SAH) on CT scan

1	No SAH on CT
2	<1 mm thick (vertical plane)
3	>1 mm thick or localized subarachnoid clot, highest rate of vasospasm
4	ICH or IVH

Abbreviations: ICH, intracerebral hemorrhage; IVH, intraventricular hemorrhage.

Table 24. Simpson grading of meningioma resection

I	Complete removal + dural resection
II	Complete removal + dural coagulation
III	Complete removal + dura left
IV	Subtotal resection
V	Simple decompression +/– biopsy

Table 25. Clinoidal meningioma grades

I	Inferior, attached to ICA
II	Arachnoid plane with ICA and optic n
III	Medial, attaches to optic n

Source: Al-Mefty O. Clinoidal meningiomas. J Neurosurg. 1990 Dec;73(6):840-849.

Table 26. Grading of vestibular schwannomas

I	Intracanalicular
II	Cisternal
III	Brain stem compression
IV	Hydrocephalus

Table 27. House–Brackmann grading for facial weakness

I	Normal	
II	Mild dysfunction	Barely noticeable
III	Moderate dysfunction	Obvious, not disfiguring
IV	Moderately severe dysfunction	Obvious, disfiguring, eyes incompletely close
V	Severe dysfunction	Barely moving
VI	Total paralysis	No movement

Source: House JW, Brackmann DE. Facial nerve grading system. *Otolaryngol Head Neck Surg* 1985 Apr;93(2):146–147

Table 28. Glomus jugulare (tympanicum) grades

A	Middle ear
B	Tympanomastoid
C	Infralabyrinthine
D	Intracranial

Table 29. Vasculitides

Vasculitis	Vessels involved	Mechanism	Pathology	Clinical Picture	Labs	Treatment
Polyarteritis nodosa (PAN)	Small and medium-sized vessels	Immune complex	Micro-aneurysms, stenosis, thrombosis, obliteration of vasa nervosum	Mononeuropathy multiplex (axonal degeneration), kidney dysfunction, necrotizing pancreatitis, purpura		Steroids, belimumab, rituximab
Systemic lupus erythematosus (SLE)	Small and large vessels	Immune complex	Inflammatory and thrombotic	Stroke, myelopathy, peripheral neuropathy, coagulopathy, Libman–Sacks endocarditis, malar butterfly rash	Antinuclear antibody (ANA), antiphospholipid antibody	
Allergic angiitis (Churg–Strauss syndrome)	Panangiitis	Immune complex		Asthma, liver failure, peripheral neuropathy, strokes, seizures, confusion	Blood eosinophilia, hematuria, albuminuria	
Serum sickness		Immune complex	PMN (polymorphonuclear leukocytes)	Fever, rash, arthritis, neuropathy, encephalomyelitis		
Temporal arteritis	External carotid artery, ophthalmic a, posterior ciliary aa	Cell-mediated	Giant cell arteritis (all three layers involved)	Elderly (70s), headache, jaw pain, shoulder pain, blindness, fever, weight loss, polymyalgia rheumatica, claudication with chewing	Increased ESR, temporal a biopsy	Steroids until ESR normalizes
Takayasu's arteritis	Aorta, pulmonary a	Cell-mediated	Giant cell arteritis, aneurysms, stenosis	Young oriental females, visual loss, loss of peripheral pulses	Increased ESR	
Wegener's granulomatosis	Intracranial, respiratory, renal	Cell-mediated		Adult males, cranial neuropathies, peripheral neuropathy	Anti-neutrophil antibodies	Steroids, Cyclophosphamide
Kawasaki's disease	Medium-sized arteries		Aneurysms, fusiform ectasia	Children, mucocutaneous lymph node syndrome		
Buerger's disease (thrombangiitis obliterans)	Small and medium-sized vessels		Thrombosis & recanalization	Tobacco, claudication, rest pain, ulcer, gangrene		
Behçet's disease	Small vessels (venules)		Arterial occlusion, aneurysm, thrombophlebitis	Males, meningo-encephalitis, brain stem edema, confusion, oro-genital ulcers, uveitis, ulcerative colitis, erythema nodosum, polyarthritis		Steroids
Cogan's syndrome	Large and medium-sized vessels			Headache, encephalitis, cavernous sinus thrombosis, strokes, peripheral neuropathy, hearing loss, Ménière's, interstitial keratitis		Steroids

Table 30. Toxicities

Toxin	Clinical Picture	Pathology	Imaging	Treatment
CO	Headache (25% Hb saturation), confusion (45%), seizures/coma (55%), dysrhythmia/death (>70%)	Bilateral hemorrhagic necrosis GPi, **cherry-red** brain	Bilateral hypodense (CT), or hypointense (MRI) GP	Oxygen, hyperbaric
CN	Respiratory failure, seizures, death	Binds cytochrome oxidase	Edema, SAH	Nitrites, thiosulfate, oxygen
ETOH	Peripheral neuropathy, myopathy, strokes, CPM, brain atrophy, cardiomyopathy, infections, death (serum ETOH > 450 mg/dL)	Demyelination, necrosis (CPM)		
	Marchiafava–Bignami disease	Corpus callosum degeneration		
	Wernicke's encephalopathy: Acute, ataxia, nystagmus, confusion, dysconjugate gaze, lateral rectus palsy, hypothermia, hypotension, coma, death (17%)	Brown–gray discoloration, loss of Purkinje cells, mammillary bodies, superior vermis, floor of 4th ventricle, periaqueductal gray, periventricular thalamus and hypothalamus	Edema, hemorrhage, demyelination, necrosis Increased serum pyruvate and thymidine tri-phosphate, decreased transketolase	Thiamine 50 mg IV
	Korsakoff's psychosis: Chronic, decreased short-term memory and learning	MD nucleus of thalamus, decreased serotonin		
	Withdrawal: seizures (1 d), tremors (1–2 ds), hallucinations and illusions (1–2 ds), delirium tremens (2–4 ds), insomnia, increased heart rate and temperature, mydriasis, sweating, death (5–15%)			Chlordiazepoxide or diazepam
	Fetal alcohol syndrome: hydrocephalus, seizures, mental retardation, cerebellar dysfunction, short palpebral fissures, epicanthal folds, low nasal bridge, short upturned nose, hypo-plastic upper lip, cleft palate, microcephaly, short stature	Neural tube defects, visceral malformation	Schizencephaly, callosal agenesis, heterotopias	
Methanol	Edema, high anion gap acidosis, vomiting, blindness (4 mL), death (100 mL) [due to formaldehyde accumulation]	Necrosis of putamen and claus-trum, optic disc swelling		Ethanol (saturates alcohol dehydroge-nase and decreases formaldehyde)
Ethylene glycol (anti-freeze)	Edema, acidosis, death (100 mL) [formation of glycolaldehyde]	Ca-oxalate in blood vessels, kidney, and brain		Ethanol
Isopropyl alcohol	Death (250 mL)			

Table 30. Toxicities (*Continued*)

Toxin	Clinical Picture	Pathology	Imaging	Treatment
Hexachlorophene (germicide)	Peripheral neuropathy (demyelination)	Spongiform degeneration of white matter		
Opiates	Hypothermia, respiratory depression, miosis, constipation, urinary retention, spasm of sphincter of Oddi, pancreatitis, pruritus **Withdrawal**: 16 hrs: lacrimation, rhinorrhea, sweating, insomnia, mydriasis, twitches, cold/hot flushes; 36 hrs: diarrhea; 72 hrs: peak			Narcan (Naloxone) 0.7 mg IV q 2 hrs Methadone 10–20 mg twice a day
Phenothiazines (chlorpromazine, prochlorperazine)	Parkinsonism (3 wks) Mental status change, seizures, orthostatic hypotension	Cholestatic jaundice, agranulocytosis		Benztropine
	Dystonia and dyskinesia			Benadryl or amantadine
	Tardive dyskinesia, akathisia			Propranolol
	Neuroleptic malignant syndrome: hyperthermia, rigidity, autonomic instability, stupor, catatonia, death (20%)	Increased CK		Dantrolene, bromocriptine
Amphetamines	Hallucination, increased respiratory rate, increased blood pressure, decreased appetite	Vasculitis	SAH	
MAO inhibitors	Increased heart rate, hypertension especially with tyramine, cheese, red wine, beer			
Tricyclic antidepressants	Urine retention, orthostatic hypotension, insomnia, agitation			Phenothiazine
Lithium	Ataxia, tremors, nystagmus, coma	Nephrogenic diabetes insipidus		
Methotrexate (especially with radiation)	Subacute necrotizing leukoencephalitis (SNLE), meningitis, encephalitis, transverse myelitis, stroke [folate antagonist]	Coagulative necrosis, lipid-laden macrophages, mineralizing angiopathy of gray matter	Bilateral symmetric demyelinating lesions	
BCNU (Gliadel) (Nitrosourea)	Necrotizing encephalomyelopathy (NEM)	Axonal swelling, arterial obliteration		
Cisplatin	Hearing loss, visual loss, peripheral neuropathy (sensory and autonomic)	Affects microtubules		
Vincristine & Vinblastine	Peripheral neuropathy (axonal degeneration)	Impaired microtubule formation		
Procarbazine	Mood changes			

(*Continued*)

Table 30. Toxicities (*Continued*)

Toxin	Clinical Picture	Pathology	Imaging	Treatment
Actinomycin D	Peripheral neuropathy	Defective transcription		
Dinitrophenol	Peripheral neuropathy	Impaired oxidative phosphorylation		
Penicillamine	Myopathy			
Tryptophan	Myopathy			
As (insecticide)	Encephalopathy, peripheral neuropathy, cardiomyopathy, shock, **Mees' lines** (transverse white lines on finger nails), increased pigmentation and hyperkeratosis of palms and soles, abdominal pain, nausea, vomiting, and diarrhea	Pancytopenia, As in urine and hair		BAL
Au	Peripheral neuropathy (axonal)			BAL, EDTA, penicillamine
Pb	Encephalitis in children: irritability, seizures, ataxia, increased ICP, coma. Abdominal pain, interstitial nephritis. Peripheral neuropathy in adults: motor only with wrist drop, demyelinating	**Basophilic stippling** of RBCs, anemia, increased blood lead level (BLL) and erythrocyte protoporphyrin, gingival Pb line, metaphyseal Pb line, increased urinary coproporphyrin III and δ-aminolevulinic acid		DMSA, penicillamine, BAL, EDTA
Hg (contaminated fish, hat dyes)	Cerebellar dysfunction, tremors, psychological problems, peripheral neuropathy, renal tubular necrosis, gastrointestinal disturbance	Defective translation, cerebellar granular layer		DMPS, DMSA, penicillamine, BAL, EDTA
Mn (miners)	Parkinsonian symptoms, psychological dysfunction, headache, pulmonary fibrosis, liver cirrhosis	Neuronal loss and gliosis in the pallidum and striatum		L-DOPA
Al	Dementia, seizures, myoclonus, pulmonary fibrosis, constipation			Deferoxamine
Thallium	Dementia, delirium, seizures, coma, peripheral neuropathy, diplopia, alopecia, cardiac dysfunction, pulmonary edema, nephritis, gastrointestinal disturbance			Prussian blue, KCl

Abbreviations: Al, aluminum; As, arsenic; Au, gold; BAL, British anti-lewisite; BCNU, bis-chloroethylnitrosourea; Ca, calcium; CN, cyanide; CO, carbon monoxide; CPM, central pontine myelinolysis; Dimercaprol, 2,3-dimercapto-propanol; DMPS, 2,3-dimercapto-1-propane-sulfonic acid; DMSA, 2,3-dimercapto-succinic acid; EDTA, ethylenediaminetetraacetic acid; Hb, hemoglobin; Hg, mercury; ETOH, alcohol; KCl, potassium chloride; L-DOPA, levo-dihydroxy-phenyl-alanine; MAO, monoamine oxidase; MD, medial dorsal; Mn, manganese; Pb, lead; SAH, subarachnoid hemorrhage.

Table 31. Anesthetics and their mechanism of action

Anesthetic	Mechanism
Isoflurane	$GABA_A$ & Glycine +
Enflurane	$GABA_A$ & Glycine +
Thiopental	$GABA_A$ +
Etomidate	$GABA_A$ +
Lidocaine	Na^+ channel blocker
Fentanyl	Opioid agonist
Ketamine	NMDA antagonist

Table 32. Common causes of hyponatremia

	CSWS	SIADH
Serum Na	Low	Low
Blood volume	Hypovolemia	Normo or hypervolemia
Serum osmolality	Normo-osmolality	Hypo-osmolality
Serum uric acid	Normal	Decreased
Urine Na	Very high	High
FeNa	High	Normal
Urine output	Polyuria	Oliguria
Urine osmolality	Increased	Increased
Treatment	Na and fluid replacement	Fluid restriction

Source: Tisdall M, Crocker M, Watkiss J, Smith M. Disturbances of sodium in critically ill adult neurologic patients: a clinical review. *J Neurosurg Anesthesiol* 2006 Jan;18(1):57–63.

Note: Rapid correction can lead to osmotic demyelination syndrome (formerly central pontine myelinolysis).

Abbreviations: CSWS, cerebral salt wasting syndrome; SIADH, syndrome of inappropriate antidiuretic hormone secretion; FeNa, fractional excretion of Na.

Table 33. Important vaso-active drugs

Drug	Chronotropic (β_1)	Inotropic (β_1)	Vasoconstrictor (α_1)	Vasodilator (β_2)
Dopamine	++	++	++ (high dose)	++ (low dose; also dopamine receptors)
Dobutamine	+	**++++**	+	++
Epinephrine	++++	++++	++++	+++
Norepinephrine (Levophed)	++	++	**++++**	+
Phenylephrine (Neosynephrine)	NO	NO	**++++**	NO
Isoproterenol	++++	++++	NO	++++

Source: Lokhandwala MF, Barrett RJ. Cardiovascular dopamine receptors: physiological, pharmacological and therapeutic implications. *J Auton Pharmacol* 1982 Sep;2(3):189–215.

Note: Bipyridines (amrinone and milrinone) are positive inotropics and vasodilators through a direct phosphodiesterase inhibitor effect (non-adrenergic) → increase cAMP → increase Ca^{++} influx. Drugs used in hypertensive emergencies: Nicardipine is a Ca^{++} channel blocker → vasodilatation → reduces blood pressure. Nitroprusside also reduces blood pressure (through nitric oxide) but may increase intracranial pressure and cause cyanide toxicity. Labetalol is α_1, β_1 and β_2 blocker → vasodilatation.

Table 34. Common antiepileptic drugs

Drug	Mechanism	Indications	Side effects	Interactions
Barbiturates	+ GABA$_A$	Generalized TC, status	Lethargy, nystagmus, ataxia, hypotension, porphyria: peripheral neuropathy and hematuria	Chloramphenicol increases barbiturates. Barbiturates decrease Coumadin.
Benzodiazepines	+ GABA$_A$	Status (of choice)	Hypotension, respiratory depression	
Propofol	+ GABA$_A$	Status (refractory)	Hypotension, respiratory depression, increased triglycerides, pancreatitis, increased risk of infection	
Phenytoin (Dilantin)	– Na$^+$ channel	Generalized TC, status (with other therapies)	Rash, Stevens–Johnson syndrome, cerebellar degeneration (ataxia, nystagmus), diplopia, stupor, peripheral neuropathy, thrombocytopenia, megaloblastic anemia, lymphadenopathy, gum hyperplasia, hirsutism, hepatitis, GI irritation, osteopenia, teratogenic (congenital fetal hydantoin syndrome)	Dilantin initially increases Coumadin (displaces from plasma proteins), long term decreases Coumadin (liver stimulation). All hepatic inhibitors increase Dilantin level (e.g., Bactrim, benzodiazepines, Coumadin). All hepatic stimulants decrease Dilantin level (e.g., barbiturates, carbamazepine). Aspirin may increase Dilantin level by displacing it from plasma proteins
Carbamazepine (Tegretol)	– Na$^+$ channel	Generalized TC	Stevens–Johnson syndrome, diplopia, nystagmus, ataxia, choreo-athetosis, pancytopenia, hyponatremia, GI irritation, toxic hepatitis (epoxycarbamazepine), oligozoospermia, teratogenic (myelomeningocele)	Erythromycin increases carbamazepine (by inhibiting its catabolism)
Lamotrigine	– Na$^+$ channel	Generalized TC, absence, Lennox–Gastaut	Blurred vision, diplopia, unsteady gait, rash, hyponatremia	
Zonisamide	– Na$^+$ channel	Generalized TC, absence	Depression, irritability, loss of appetite, weakness	
Valproate	Increased GABA, – Na$^+$ channel, – Ca^{++} channel	Absence, complex partial, generalized TC, myoclonus	Hepatotoxic, tremors, polycystic ovaries, oligozoospermia, small testicles, teratogenic (myelomeningocele), hyponatremia	Valproate increases level of Dilantin, phenobarbital, and lamotrigine. Aspirin may increase valproate level by displacing it from plasma proteins
Topiramate	+ GABA$_A$, – Na$^+$ channel, – Ca^{++} channel	Generalized TC, Lennox–Gastaut, headache	Drowsiness, weakness, mood changes	

Table 34. Common antiepileptic drugs

Felbamate	– NMDA, + GABA	Generalized TC, Lennox–Gastaut	Aplastic anemia, liver failure, anorexia, insomnia
Ethosuximide	– Ca⁺⁺ channel	Absence	Choreo-athetosis, GI irritation
Levetiracetam (Keppra)	– Synaptic vesicle protein 2A (SV2A)	Generalized TC	Drowsiness, weakness, mood changes (irritability)
ACTH	– CRH, (+ melanocortin receptors)	West syndrome (infantile spasms)	Infections

Abbreviations: ACTH, adrenocorticotropic hormone; CRH, corticotropin-releasing hormone; GI, gastrointestinal; TC, tonic–clonic; +, stimulates; –, inhibits.

Source: Henschel O, Gipson KE, Bordey A. GABAA receptors, anesthetics and anticonvulsants in brain development. *CNS Neurol Disord Drug Targets* 2008 Apr;7(2):211–224; Patsalos PN, Fröscher W, Pisani F, van Rijn CM. The importance of drug interactions in epilepsy therapy. *Epilepsia* 2002 Apr; 43(4):365–385

Book References

Andrews BT. *Intensive Care in Neurosurgery*. New York, NY: AANS, Thieme; 2003

Burt AM. *Textbook of Neuroanatomy*. Philadelphia, PA: WB Saunders; 1993

Carpenter MB. *Core Text of Neuroanatomy*. 4th ed. Baltimore, MD: Williams & Wilkins; 1991

Citow JS, Macdonald RL, Kraig RP, Wollmann RL, eds. *Comprehensive Neurosurgery Board Review*. New York, NY: Thieme; 2000

Ellison D, Love S, Chimelli L, Harding BN, Lowe J, Vinters HV, eds. *Neuropathology: A Reference Text of CNS Pathology*. 2nd ed. Edinburgh, UK: Mosby, Elsevier; 2004

Hanna A. *Anatomy and Exposures of Spinal Nerves*. Switzerland: Springer; 2015

Hanna A. *Nerve Cases*. Switzerland: Springer; 2017

Marino PL. *The ICU Book*. 2nd ed. New York, NY: Lippincott Williams & Wilkins; 1998

Rhoton AL. *Cranial Anatomy and Surgical Approaches*. New York, NY: Neurosurgery, Lippincott Williams & Wilkins; 2003

Squire LR, Bloom FE, McConnell SK, Roberts JL, Spitzer NC, Zigmond MJ, eds. *Fundamental Neuroscience*. 2nd ed. San Diego, CA: Academic Press, Elsevier; 2003

Williams PL, Warwick R, eds. *Gray's Anatomy*. 36th ed. London, UK: Churchill Livingstone; 1980

Woolsey TA, Hanaway J, Gado MH, eds. *The Brain Atlas: A Visual Guide to the Human Central Nervous System*. 2nd ed. Hoboken, NJ: Wiley; 2003

Index

Note: Page numbers set italic indicate figures or tables.